SOS
EXERCISE-
SCHMEXERCISE

SOS
EXERCISE-SCHMEXERCISE

THE EFFORTLESS WEIGHT-LOSS AND HEALTH SOLUTION WITH THE TROPICAL TURBO METABOLISM PLAN

NO EXERCISE NOR CALORIE COUNTING NECESSARY

KATHARINA BACHMAN

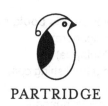

PARTRIDGE

To order additional copies of this book, contact
Toll Free 800 101 2657 (Singapore)
Toll Free 1 800 81 7340 (Malaysia)
orders.singapore@partridgepublishing.com

www.partridgepublishing.com/singapore

Preliminary Notes

Forget about all the diets known to humanity so far! Kiss your over-weight and consequent diseases, and even your cellulite good-bye for good!

By using the new »SOS - Exercise-Schmexercise«, The Effortless Weight Loss and Health Solution Plan, Germany has lost over a million pounds – with no yo-yo-effect! But even better: no more high blood pressure, no more high cholesterol, allergies, autoimmune diseases, and no more diabetes. German globetrotter and Author Katharina Bachman, at home in Asia, was extremely fortunate when fate led her to Indian Dr. K.S. in Kuala Lumpur. His expertise and vast experience turned her and her husband into new, happy and healthy people! A seven-day detox-program, followed by a customized nutrition plan, showed them the path to a brand new life. Hundreds of thousands of people in Germany, Austria and Switzerland now follow this path.

Written in her refreshingly open and witty style, the author's bestseller is the story of her life's greatest miracle. Sold out within hours of publication, its first edition sales sky-rocketed in German-speaking countries to 100,000 copies in just nine months, »SOS - Exercise-Schmexercise« continues to be a phenomenal success. Facebook is overflowing with thousands of testimonials from happy people about their achievements and their trust in the successful SOS-Method. SOS now stands for a brand new and successful life-style philosophy. It is thanks to Katharina Bachman's success, that many exotic superfoods are available in most supermarkets in Germany today.

Detox. Lose weight. Be healthy and happy. Jump on it!

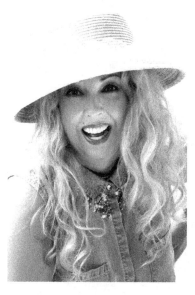

KATHARINA BACHMAN is a good 30 pounds overweight, suffers from the various ailments known in our western industrial world and takes a daily arsenal of medications when she walks into Dr. K.S.' practice in 2013. The Indian doctor prescribes a detoxification plan and subsequent transformative tropical power-food diet. Her excess pounds melt away at record speed. Her diabetes disappears and her blood pressure is stabilized. Even her loathsome cellulite vanishes …

In this book, Katharina Bachman not only tells her own success story, but shares her newfound knowledge on the subject with the world. By embracing her highly effective plan to balance your metabolism, you can feast on tropical culinary delights while simultaneously losing excess weight in a healthy manner.

Preamble

A small part of the German media was reluctant to feature my book, because of its title "Schlank ohne Sport" – the English translation of which is "Slim without Sports", whereas "sports", in this case, refers to physical exercising for fitness and not sports as a game or team activity. Without having read it, the media found the title to suggest the book's content to be anti-sports, as in the latter context mentioned above. This is by no means the case.

This book merely focuses on my personal story, about how I was able to regain a slim figure without exercising, and, in the process, overcome an array of illnesses.

Nevertheless, we should also take into account the many people unable to partake in athletic activity, due to severe accidents, to being confined to a wheelchair, or other serious illnesses preventing exercise.

Let us also consider the countless mothers, having to take care of three, four or five family members; and all the single mothers, some of whom have two or three jobs to make ends meet.

Not to mention the large number of people with highly stressful jobs requiring frequent international travel who simply have no time to exercise regularly. And then there are the people, such as myself, who abhor exercising and find going to the gym just plain torturous.

This book is neither a guideline for avoiding sports or exercise, nor does it promote a sedentary life-style without exercising for fitness. On the contrary! However, while some people may not have the time, others may lack the inclination, and yet others are simply not able to exercise on a regular basis. Should these people remain overweight, or worse, obese, and consequently become ill? No, in my opinion, not at all!

A Short Introduction

Forget about all the diets known to humanity so far and kiss your over-weight and your cellulite good-bye!

This book tells you how an Indian doctor in Malaysia guided my husband and me back to being slim, fit and most importantly, healthy in a very short period of time. This "miracle" is not attributed to any mysterious magic pill or potion, but to ancient Indian, Mayan and Aztec wisdom. We have been happy and content again ever since, enjoying our new exciting life. We're convinced that you too, can experience the same miracle!

CONTENTS

PART I

PART II

Katharina's Coconut Deodorant - Bath Oil - Vegetable Soup - Baking Powder - Coconut Oil - Coconut Milk - Coconut Cream - Coconut Butter - Almond Milk (Almond Milk, Unflavoured) - Vanilla Flavored Almond Milk - Cinnamon Flavored Almond Milk - Coconut Almond Milk - Pandan Essence - Maybe Butter - Tomato Butter - Mushroom Butter - Honey Substitute - Chocolate

*"The Exterior of a Plant is
merely half of its reality."*

JOHANN WOLFGANG VON GOETHE (1799)

PART I

Let the Transformation Begin ...

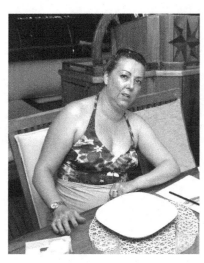
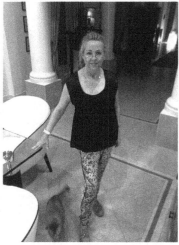

Preface

Admittedly, the title of this book sounds provocative because losing weight without exercising is by no means desirable for everyone, nor is it necessarily healthy from a medical point of view. But in the following, you will find out how we - that is, my husband and I - succeeded in doing so despite all odds. The catchy title was aimed at enticing you - yes, you, dear reader! - to buy this book. Which, apparently, I have managed to do.

The reason is simple: I wish to make money. This may disappoint, or even shock you. However, there is no need for that, since it is only part of the whole truth. Of course I want to profit, among other things, by my efforts. Who wouldn't? The rest of the truth, however, is far more important for you personally! I would like to share with you the wonderful feeling of losing many pounds within a short time, so that you also can experience it. My success story can become your success story. If you want it to.

First of all, I am not telling my story as a medical doctor, but as a writer. I want to share with you, in detail, how my husband and I each lost over 24 pounds (!) in three months, simultaneously detoxifying our bodies in the process - in my case, without any exercise at all. Besides having lost all those excess pounds, I found especially gratifying that my cellulite had suddenly vanished as well! Along with the undeniable health benefits, for me, this was the proverbial "cherry on top".

The sole purpose of this book is to answer the question: How on earth did my husband and I manage to lose weight, get back into good shape and become completely healthy in such a short time?

We all know the problem: Almost everyone feels more or less over-weight, or is, in fact, too heavy. A recent study by the Oxford University confirms that 64 percent of all men and 49 percent of all women in Germany are over-weight - world-wide, a total of 2.1 billion people are affected. And the number is steadily, rapidly, and inexorably growing. Diseases such as diabetes, high blood pressure, heart problems, including heart attacks, and cancer are the devastating consequences. Obesity not only burdens the people suffering from it, it also affects our entire health care system. Time is of the essence for governments to face the challenge of finding a solution to the problem. The huge increase in treatment costs for being over-weight and associated illnesses and side-effects is projected to double in the next ten years. So let's get started! It's really not that hard. The 7-Day Detox Plan is the first step in achieving sustained weight-loss and counteracting all these diseases. There is no yo-yo effect. We too, were victims of all the consequences of a bad, unhealthy diet. For years, we were taking an endless array of medications for our ailments. Until the day my husband came down with a bad cold …

Before starting with Doctor K.S.'s program, I was extremely skeptical. In the past 20 years, we had tried several slimming cures and diets, breaking some of them off, following through with others. Yet none kept their promise, and when there were any results, they were middling and short-lived. On top of that, I found calorie counting really annoying, the same as constantly having to watch my figure, exercise, and all the rest of it. I was frankly sick and tired of having to give up this, that and the other thing - all this never ending self-torture and the requirement to exercise, exercise, exercise. I simply hate exercising! Always have. So, if you're imagining the proverbial couch potato, that's me! That is why I especially admire all those people dutifully jogging and gladly hitting the gym with vigor and enthusiasm.

I had resigned myself to the fact that, after a certain age, it was normal not to have jeans, skirts and t-shirts in size S in my closet - not to mention XS - and that my clothes would come in circus-tent sizes from now on.

And at my age, I no longer had much interest in looking like Twiggy anymore anyway. All told, I had come to terms with obesity, overweight, high blood pressure, diabetes, high cholesterol and shortness of breath when climbing stairs etc. I never dreamed I could ever go back to wearing a size 10, having a decent figure and normal blood pressure, sugar, and cholesterol readings, or that my ever swollen belly would disappear. So - aren't you curious now about all that I have to tell you?

At this point, I would like to thank you very much for buying my book. The small price you have paid will help repay the cost of Doctor K.S.'s program. I must say, getting my health back and slimming down turned out to be fairly expensive, especially because, among other purchases, I needed a completely new wardrobe, along with several new pairs of shoes - mine had all become too large! And everyone knows what a big deal *buying shoes* is for us women, right?

Now, once you have successfully lost weight, please tell all your family, friends, colleagues, neighbors and anyone else you can think of to read this book.

I wish you great success from the bottom of my heart.

Katharina Bachman

PS: This is to be regarded as a guideline and inspiration, rather than a set of unpleasant instructions - it should give you courage and enthusiasm for a new beginning!

Coincidence or Fate?

Often a mere coincidence can cause big changes in our lives, even if we don't grasp their impact until much later. In fact, usually, things appear to be quite harmless, and so it was with us. My husband had caught a bad cold and wanted to see a doctor. Feeling low and not wanting to endure the torture of heavy traffic, he looked for one in our neighborhood. He soon found a small doctor's office right around the corner. I should explain that, at this point, we had recently moved back to Kuala Lumpur after having lived in Dubai for some time. We were familiar with the teeming city from the time we lived in Malaysia for six years. So we knew it would take at least two hours to reach the city center. Having a doctor nearby is always a good idea. Also, we felt that any general practitioner could help my husband with a common cold. So he went to the small office around the corner.

During the course of the consultation, the lady doctor made a pretty nasty remark: "You are too fat, you have to go on a diet." She advised my husband to see a specialist. And lo and behold, she knew of just such a specialist, right there in the building, only one floor up. My husband came home with some cold medication and told me all about his hurtful "You are too fat" encounter. Driven by curiosity, and also perhaps due to the pretty lady doctor's drastic remark, he did, in fact, end up going to said specialist a few weeks later. From then on, our lives changed dramatically.

A Turbaned Indian Physician: Dr. K.S.

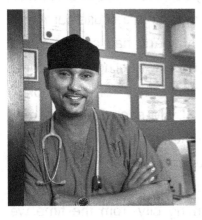 Going in to my first appointment, I had serious doubts. I thought it was all hocus-pocus, if not an outright scam. As it turned out, the specialist just happened to be the pretty lady doctor's very own brother, Doctor K. S., an Indian physician, wearing a black turban. He was a member of the Sikh religious community. The copious amounts of herbal concoctions he prescribed to take daily were not exactly a bargain. Nevertheless, my better half started the detoxification program. I however, wanted to see positive results first and preferred waiting for the time being.

Only four days later, I found myself in his office, urgently requesting an appointment, which I was granted for the next day. The examination began with an extensive blood analysis. The doctor took blood samples in the morning before breakfast and after 6 in the evening. The microbiological analysis took an entire week - the time necessary for various cultures to develop.

Next came my first consultation, which lasted a full two hours. I was shocked by the results. For several years, up to this point in my life, I had been on multiple medications for high blood pressure, diabetes, high cholesterol and a severe allergy. I was using a cortisone based asthma inhaler and ingesting thyroid hormones - as you can see, enough to stock small pharmacy. My doctors in both Germany and Dubai told me in no uncertain terms, that I would be taking all these pills for the rest of my life. With this wonderful prognosis, I fell into temporary depression, which led to yet further medication.

Here I was in Dr. K.S.' office, listening to this detailed explanation of my hair-raising blood test results, feeling worse and worse by the minute.

Oh, my God! This is a disaster. I am deathly ill. I will surely have a heart attack or a stroke. It won't be long now. This is the end!

A hurricane of terrifying thoughts started forming in my mind, with pitch black clouds and blinding flashes of lightening tearing through my brain.

At this point, the doctor's words reached me only through a dense fog. I felt anger rising. Tremendous anger. I did not like Dr. K.S. - of that I was becoming increasingly certain.

I already knew all that. So what are you going to do about it? Know-it-all.

"You must lose weight, lose your body fat, and detoxify immediately", he kept repeating, and "exercise! Go to the gym! Twice a week at least." At this point I could have strangled him with my bare hands.

Hallelujah. I hate exercise - exercise - exercise!

Obviously, yours truly knows exactly how important every day exercise is for good health. But please let me make this short and sweet: I'm. Just. Too. Lazy!

While Dr. K.S. kept talking on and on, I was feeling worse and worse. And suddenly I heard the words "repair", "good results", and "guaranteed".

"Repair?", I asked, surprised and becoming curious.

"Yes, first we will fix your kidneys and your liver", he answered enthusiastically, as though he were planning a fun birthday party. He explained how ailing organs "communicated" with each other, and which effects taking one or the other medication would have on them. For example, cholesterol lowering medication can lead to poor liver test values.

In other words, the various pills for diabetes and high blood pressure I was ingesting on a daily basis were, in turn, attacking my kidneys and my liver. As a result, in the near future, this would cause one or more new health problems, for which I would need yet further medication and so on and so forth. The Indian "Doc" described to me, in great detail, how he was going to "repair" all this. He was quite knowledgeable, at least as far as I could tell. Nevertheless, I still did not like him one bit better.

To begin with, he wanted me to start with his special detoxification plan, which he described as "very efficient". Once at home, having read through the two-page instructions, I found them surprisingly easy to carry out.

BY THE WAY: About the Sikh Turban
During my sessions with Dr. K.S., we also came upon the subject of his turban, which has played an important role in Indian culture for thousands of years. In early times, rulers wore splendidly ornate turbans as a symbol of their authority and nobility. Still today, at traditional weddings, Indian men of all religions wear turbans. The size, shape and color are indicative of the wearer's region and culture.

The Sikh turban, known as "Dastar", is not a purely cultural headdress. It also has a religious and spiritual significance. A Sikh becomes one, so to speak, with his turban. He considers it part of his head. The Sikh turban, including the splendid head of hair it covers, carries deep traditional meaning; the baptized Sikh takes an oath to preserve all of his hair, never to cut it, and to adorn it with a turban for the rest of his life. For a Sikh, preserving his hair is an expression of simplicity, humility and dignity: the turban symbolizes an inner attitude showing the wearer's dignity, commitment, self-respect, courage and religious devotion. He wears it out of love, a profound sense of duty, and respect for, and according to his belief in the the Sikh prophet.

The daily twenty-minute ritual of tying the turban is performed with devotion and reverence, much like a true work of art. It requires a certain dexterity to master the thin, seven-meter long, by one meter wide, cotton cloth.

Before tying the turban, Sikhs twist their hair into a bun, covering it with a hair net, as a sort of under-turban. When a Sikh leaves the house, he wears his "main turban" which covers the bun while forming an open pyramid shape on his forehead.

Sikhs remain Sikhs for the duration of their lives. While only those living holistically, truthfully and consciously, in harmony with themselves and remaining true to the deeper purpose of their lives deserve to be held in high esteem.

Women also sometimes wear turbans, however this has nothing to do with covering their hair for the purpose of hiding it from the gaze of others, as is the case in Islam. For Sikh women, it is rather a way of dressing up. But generally, women wanting to cover their head, simply wear a thin cotton headscarf.

Getting Started is Easy

Dr. K.S.' regimen began on a Monday morning, rather simply, with a seven-day detoxification. My husband had already successfully completed his first week, but out of love for me, (or at least I hope so,) and because he wished to lose some more weight, he started over again with me.

We were to weigh ourselves every morning after waking up and write down the (at this point aggravating) results. Accordingly, we kept meticulous weight records. I diligently typed our respective weights into my smart phone day after day. To avoid the daily jostling for the single set of scales in our home, we bought a second one, placing it right next to the one we already had.

At the beginning of our transformation in August 2013, my scales displayed a nasty 151.6 pounds, at a *scant* height of 5'2". At the time I was wearing clothes size XXL, and heading toward a size 16.

My husband's scales were even more cruel: At a height of 5'6", the display ruthlessly showed 234.1 pounds. Woah! His pants were a size 38, in other words XXL. His belts showed an impressive 3'7" and his shirt size was also a proud 38, with a collar size 18.

All in all, there were plenty of good reasons for us to slim down.

After the first detox day, I had, believe it or not, actually lost 2.2 pounds. Full of anticipation, I stepped on the scales on day two: A total of 3.5 pounds less since day one. Not bad.

By day three, I weighed 146.6. I had lost a little over 0.7 pounds. Not so great.

Day four was a minus of 0.9 pounds.

Day five was rather disappointing again. I had lost only another 0.7 pounds - weighing a total of 144.2 pounds.

On day six, I had cause to celebrate: I had gone down another 1.8 pounds.

After seven days, I weighed 142.6 pounds, which means I had lost a grand total of 9 pounds in a week!

And, in case you are wondering, today I weigh 119 pounds and so have lost over 31 pounds in total. My better half achieved a somewhat higher score, but then again, he was a lot chubbier than I was to begin with. (Sorry, darling). Today he weighs 180 pounds and buys his T-shirts in men's size S.

In the following, I will explain in detail just how we did it. And, in my case, without any exercise whatsoever.

Easy - Going - Our First Successes

We had accomplished our seven day plan. I was truly surprised at having lost over 9 pounds in such a short time - and all without painful food cravings nor feeling deprived. It was really an easy-peasy detox plan. I conceded that Dr. K.S. had earned half a brownie point. But he still had a ways to go on the "I - like - and - trust - you" scale - because in my book, he was still at minus ten points because of the dollar signs I continued to imagine seeing in his eyes. This feeling was doubled because of the huge amounts of very expensive natural remedies we were required to ingest - a large box for each of us. Tons of pills, to be taken morning, noon, and night; all hand-sorted, bagged and tagged according to BB (before breakfast), AB (after breakfast), BD (before dinner) and AD (after dinner), another pill at 11 AM and one before going to sleep.

Whether vitamin products and dietary supplements are necessary or not has been a subject of discussion for some time now.

The specific use of vitamins, minerals and trace elements primarily serves to supplement the ones actually missing in our systems. Be sure to have a doctor you trust perform the necessary lab tests before buying anything you might "think" you need. The targeted intake of certain vitamins supports our immune system, our bones, and keeps our organs healthy. This is especially important during a dietary regimen.

People living on a balanced diet rarely need any vitamins whatsoever. Unfortunately, most of us don't manage a perfectly healthy diet. And at certain times, depending on the season or during pregnancy, our food does not supply us with sufficient nutrients. Today nutrition societies recommend taking dietary supplements to fill certain "gaps".

At our first appointment after the detoxification, Dr. K.S. gave us high praise for our perseverance. He said he could not say the same for his Asian patients, most of them never came back. "You Germans are so conscientious. You can be always be relied upon", he commended us - probably aiming to sell us further loads of boxes full of vitamin pills.

"And now the time has come for a rigorous change in diet, according to blood type," he added quickly, blitzing us with reams of documents describing everything about blood type specific nutrition and PH-balance. For each of us, he had compiled a customized nutrition plan, listing the various vitamins to support it, because, he added ominously, an unbalanced diet was the greatest evil of all. But our vitamin status had already been determined during the very first blood test. We had already been told specifically which vitamins, minerals and trace elements our bodies needed. Furthermore, neither my husband nor I had ever heard of blood type diets. Once back home, we settled on our comfortable terrace to read through the documents attentively.

Oh, my God! According to this, I was to be deprived of so many of my very favorite delicacies, such as balsamic vinegar, tomatoes, meat, mangos, and the list went on. *Oh, man,* my husband groaned just seconds later. "No more red cabbage and Brussel sprouts?" But that was not the end of it. And although we kept whining and yammering, with a heavy heart, we resigned ourselves to sticking with our new nutrition list to the letter. After all, our reputation of being "dependable Germans" was on the line.

Dealing with chopping vegetables was especially tedious and on-going on a daily basis. So, to lighten things up, we would turn on the kitchen radio and listen to the babble of a German program we got via the internet. Usually the news we were hearing from our old home country got us so riled up that slicing vegetables into small pieces became less of an annoying task. And at the end of the day, we produced delicious, healthy meals, which were in perfect accordance with our blood types.

Time went by, week after week, and our excess pounds just melted away. The more weight we lost, the more enthusiastic we became about slicing and dicing. We had become accustomed to the task and even developed efficient techniques to move it along faster. And lickety-split, our meals were served. Man is, and remains, a creature of habit.

We put it to the test. Is it possible to prepare a fresh meal at home faster than - or at least just as fast as - ordering in or taking out?

We tried it one day. On your mark, get set, go! My husband jumped in the car to a fast-food place just five minutes down the street, while I prepared our meal of fresh ingredients. When he came back with a bag full of unhealthy food, I had already laid the table with a delicious fresh dinner. And at the fast-food place, there were only two people ahead of him, waiting in line for their fatal junk food. So we now had proof: preparing a fresh, home-made meal went just as quickly as picking something up from a take-out. The pizza delivery service took even longer. By the time it arrived, we had finished our dinner. Of course we didn't eat any of the terrible fast-food. And, last but not least, we were pleased to discover that home-cooking was more economical.

A New Way of Eating

In the meantime, I had many questions regarding certain aspects of his medical orders, and I felt an urgent need to communicate with Dr. K.S. In particular, his blood type diets and acid/base balance needed further clarification. For weeks, I researched the contents of his vast documentation, studying the material in conventional and alternative medical literature, as well as on the internet. As the gaps in my knowledge were closing, I felt reasonably "enlightened". Whereupon I credited Dr. K.S. with two brownie points at one go.

As to be expected, I encountered critics, such as the German Nutrition Association, opposing the so-called blood type diets. On its website, it draws scathing conclusions regarding Dr. D'Adamo's blood type diets. Among other things, it states that the diets are "seductively easy sounding assumptions" which Dr. D'Adamo advocates without any scientific evidence. Feeling very disillusioned, I needed another appointment with Dr. K.S. Usually these consultations take a good two hours. This clarifying session however was a whole new story, lasting a full 4 hours.

"Research on certain human characteristics based on their blood types originated in Japan, as early as 1916", Dr. K.S. professed. And I learned that in 1930, psychologist Professor Furukawa Takeji had published on the subject in the German scholarly journal "Zeitschrift für Angewandte

Psychologie". On the other hand, in 1957, American Dr. James D'Adamo did serious research on the connection between food compatibility and blood types. Advocates of the blood type diet have since emerged, who feel partially confirmed by current gene-research - as well as opponents - like the German Nutrition Association, which contends that Dr. D'Adamo's findings lack scientific evidence and that the diet is therefore unhealthy.

For me personally, I can say, without a doubt in my mind, that this nutrition plan was truly miraculous for my husband and myself. And let's be honest, on any given subject, there are always naysayers. It's the same with every new thing we hear or read. First something is good for us, then it's not. I remember the time when my beloved eggs for breakfast were vilified as the culprit causing high cholesterol. In the meantime, this opinion has been revised. You are about to find out just how healthy they are! Maybe moderation is the measure of all things after all. Many years ago, a very old Chinese woman told me a wise legend on moderation, which still impresses me to this day.

Here is that short Chinese legend:
A man by the name of Lee Ho had been living in a village near Suzhou for twenty-five years. One day, he could no longer bare the endless grasping for power and money, and the egotistical, self-serving ways of his fellow men. In his anger, he decided to leave his village. He went on a

quest to find peace and serenity. After days of wandering, he sat down on a mountain top overlooking the banks of the Yangtze Kiang river, swearing never to leave that spot again. From then on, he lived only on the bounty of Nature. Even though he soon noticed that this could not be the bliss he had hoped to find on his quest, he nevertheless remained on the mountain top, deep in thought. Years later, covered in bird droppings, weather beaten and nearly mummified, he happened to overhear a conversation an old Chinaman was having with his grandson. The two were gliding along the river in a junk. The grandson was playing the ukulele. What dreadful music, Lee Ho thought. "Son", he heard the grandfather say, "you must tighten them properly, you need to tighten the strings some more." The grandson did as his grandfather advised. Again, the boy tried to coax a melody from his instrument. And again, the ukulele made only screeching sounds. The grandfather looked at his grandson and said: "No, son, now you have tightened them too much. Find the true middle. You must find the balance!" Again, the boy did as his grandfather advised, and suddenly, beautiful, enchanting music poured forth. Lee Ho was as delighted as he was astonished. He pondered for a while and suddenly he knew what he had to do. He tore off the hardened crust covering his body, stood up and went back to his village near Suzhou. From then on, Lee Ho lived a balanced life of perfect moderation. He had found the peace and serenity he had been searching for so long.

20

Finding the Mean as the Measure of All Things

I will possibly be stoned for this story by an angry crowd of mental coaches, who constantly preach to their clients that the balance found in moderation equals mediocrity and is not good enough. In my opinion, constant striving for perfection is a relationship killer, makes us sick, and is the cause of all sorts of evil. Everything should always become bigger and better, higher and faster. And so it is with our eating behavior. Hurry to McDriveThru and company - no time to waste - and forget about cooking at home. Our tables are spread with fast and processed food, canned goods and deliveries. This makes us ill, fills doctors' offices and lines the pockets of the pharmaceutical industry. On the other hand, I am aware that the people working in the pharma industry are just trying to make a living, the same as the numerous doctors and employees in the medical field. If, worldwide, just 50 percent of these people had no work, it would be a catastrophe. This clearly shows that finding the mean is the measure of all things. I am the last person to want to be the judge of other people's eating habits. Nor do I condemn the pharmaceutical industry in its entirety - but it is essential for all of us to be able to lead stress-free lives and enjoy healthy nutrition.

Here the pharma industry and food producing companies alike could contribute immensely, if they were less profit-oriented. Natural remedies are not patentable, and thus of little interest to these branches of industry. Perhaps they fear that without patents, they will be vulnerable to free competition? That's just nonsense! This is about all of us, about humanity and humanity's health. If pharmaceutical companies were to produce remedies made with natural ingredients, without patents - providing the most affordable, highest quality products - they would have the opportunity to enhance their reputation and earn our approval. Critics would literally be silenced, and all of humanity would profit. Nature offers ample possibilities for healing and science is fully capable of searching nature for healing substances and employing them to keep people healthy. Countless studies of leading scientists and medical professionals back up this fact, along with just as many success stories of healing.

Medication-Free at Last!

The following step in our success story finds us at the next appointment at our Indian doctor's office. The minute he welcomed us, he showered us with compliments. I had lost another 11 pounds, and my husband 17.6 pounds. My rating of Dr. K.S. went up by another point in my book. And today, the dollar signs in his eyes seemed to have paled. Had I possibly misjudged him? Yet, I decided to wait a while before passing final judgement. We still had the next extensive blood panel ahead of us and I was not yet fully convinced of whether or not the yoyo effect might make our weight bounce right back up to where it had been.

But my fingers had become thinner, and my wedding ring was loose. And as I mentioned earlier, I even had to go out and buy new shoes. Yay! I finally had a reason to do so. Isn't that great? My toes and feet were as slim as they had been when I was twenty years old. I had lost fatty deposits that previous "normal" diets never seemed to get rid of. And regarding my feminine contours, everything was still in the right place. For me, this was a first. All the diets I tried over the past twenty years had always subjected my breasts to radical weight loss. The "super-magic-fast" diets also had the undesired effect of causing super fast weight loss in certain areas, especially my face. "You look sick", I was told. So our enthusiasm was even greater, when my husband, having recently dropped 33 pounds, now looked vibrant, healthy and handsome. We also noticed that our taste-buds had become much more sensitive. Flavors were suddenly more intense. Bread, vegetables, desserts, and meat from grass-fed animals tasted like real meat, and butter tasted like butter.

Two weeks later, we got our blood test results. With a twinkle in his eye and my results in hand, Dr. K.S. said: "Katharina, starting tomorrow, you can stop taking one of your diabetes medications."

What great news! Anyone dealing with this disease can surely imagine how I felt at that moment.

Our doc gave me "Cinsulin" (see page 81), which would now replace that medication. And for this wonderful news, he got another brownie point. His approval rating was gradually rising, and as I left his office that day, I actually started liking him just a little tiny bit. And although we had no clue whatsoever, let alone dared to consider the possibility, the day my husband and I were to be completely free of all medication was approaching quickly.

We went on living according to our doctor's nutrition plan and continued slimming down. In time, I created my own "instructions" because I did not want to have to do without certain foods - like meat - which was marked as unsuitable for my blood type. I had a simple guideline for our meals. On 300 out of the year's 365 days, we would eat according to Dr. K.S.' plan. The remaining 65 days, we would enjoy as our "Fun Days" to reward ourselves at least once a week. Well, actually 1.25 times to be exact, since a year has 52 weeks.

Six months later, my husband took the very last of his many prescription drugs. For years he had been taking countless pills for high cholesterol, elevated uric acid levels, allergies and high blood pressure, which had been, by the way, diagnosed as "hereditary" by previous doctors, who told him that he would be taking blood pressure medicine for the rest of his life.

Kissing My Diabetes Good-Bye

One day, Dr. K.S asked me: "Katharina, when you dilute three tablespoons of sugar in less than half a cup of water and drink it, it tastes terribly sweet, doesn't it?" I agreed. "So", he went on, "how can you remove the sugar from your beverage?" I looked at him quizzically, having no idea what he meant. "It's simple, you just keep adding water! For instance, a person with elevated blood sugar levels should drink a lot of water. Preferably still water at room temperature, in other words, not ice-cold." Whereupon, he launched into another one of his lengthy lectures - this time on diabetes. Looking back, after following his plan for just under a year, I saw that they now gave me a "joy" day, as my dear friend Sylke likes to say when anything wonderful happened to her. On this very day, Dr. K.S. announced exuberantly: "From now on, you no longer need any diabetes medication whatsoever. Your blood sugar levels have been normal for quite some time, and, while you're at it, you can also leave off your blood pressure pills. Consider yourself medication-free." Two days later, I began writing this book.

Doctor K.S. started by replacing my current daily diabetes medicine named Diamicron MR 60 mg, with Trajenta 5 mg, stating that the latter was generally easier on my system and not as hard on my kidneys. Shortly after, my blood sugar levels went down noticeably. Intrigued by the positive effects of this drug, I started researching it. I found out that for quite some time now, "Trajenta" was successfully being used for diabetes in the US, Japan and many other countries worldwide.

Although initially approved in Germany as well, the Gemeinsame Bundesausschuss der Ärzte, Apotheker und Krankenhäuser, (GBA) - the joint federal committee of physicians, pharmacists and hospitals - which is required to establish additional effectiveness benefits of drugs, in order to ensure health insurance coverage, retracted the approval of Trajenta in February 2013. This, of course, hurts those with public health insurance - millions of diabetes patients in Germany. Paradoxically, the drug is considered the great beacon of hope in the battle against diabetes. "The GBA decision is contrary to the very basis of medicine and science", according to Boehringer Ingelheim pharmaceutical company. "Negotiating prices with the Federal Associations of Health Insurance Funds based on additional effectiveness assessments is nonsensical. The Funds base their pricing on generic products. For an innovative and patented medication, such a price is unacceptable in Germany", comments Dr. Engelbert Günster, CEO of Boehringer Ingelheim in Germany, to leading German news weekly, *Der Spiegel*. Generic products are copies, so to speak, and cost much less. The down side is that the pharma companies, due to a lack of funding, discontinue further research and development. If, however, a new medication is not researched and developed, no generic version of said medication will be produced. Be this as it may, ten months after Dr. K.S. entered our lives, all was well with the world again. Step by step, he had replaced our current drugs with less damaging ones, moved on to exchanging these with all-natural remedies until we were finally entirely free of all chemical medication.

As I mentioned before, Dr. K.S. prescribed a cinnamon extract (Cinsulin), which I take three times daily to this day (see page 81).

Our friends overwhelmed us with compliments: *You look fantastic, so young, fit and vibrant. Your skin, your hair, amazing. You look at least ten, if not fifteen years younger.*

And that's exactly how we feel now. We are happy, content and enjoy boundless energy. But the very best occurred on a sunny day. You will soon find out what happened. In October 2011, I was still thinking, "my life is moving towards inevitable deterioration, to my sure demise". Walking was a true challenge. I was fat, sluggish and listless, and my blood levels were frightening. As you now know, I had type 2 diabetes, high blood pressure, allergies, and elevated cholesterol. My liver and kidneys were compromised, and I was suffering from all the well-known symptoms of menopause, including depression. For all of this I was taking copious amounts of medicine, most of which negatively impacted my other organs. I was just about ready to get taken out with the trash. Hallelujah.

So imagine how exhilarated I feel today, now that my life, health and wellbeing are restored.

Discovering New Foods

One day, I ran into an old acquaintance, born here in Asia, who looked *really* good, because he had just lost over twenty pounds. I had always only known Thomas as *Dicki* ("Fatty"). "Hey, you look great", I said. Three months earlier, he too had changed his way of eating - no more rice, which, as the staple food in Asia, is a real challenge. No more noodles, here mainly served as rice noodles, which made them equally difficult to avoid. No potatoes - less of a problem since Asians don't really care for them.

By leaving off only these three carb-loaded foods, Thomas had managed to lose considerable weight within just three months, simultaneously improving his health.

For us, rice and noodles are pretty much off our list; and, except on rare occasions, on a Fun Day, we hardly ever eat potatoes anymore, even though we Germans love potatoes. And when we do have them, it's always with the skin. I didn't mind leaving rice off very much. Potatoes, on the other hand, were a bigger deal, which both of us managed to overcome. I would like to emphasize, that potatoes in moderation are not really problematic from a nutritional point of view. Years ago, our healthcare practitioner in Berlin had advised us to go on a potato diet. The diet consisted of eating up to eight unpeeled (!) potatoes a day, over a period of six weeks. Some of his patients lost weight on the diet. It may be, though, that these people simply lost weight because they were so full of potatoes that their caloric intake was reduced, because they didn't fill up on anything else. In any case, eating only potatoes was not an option for us.

More often than not, most diets turn out to be mere "episodes", since they usually have the opposite effect of what is intended - sustainable weigh loss. Fat-free and low-calorie diets usually lack important proteins - those found in fish, for example - and we are left with nutrients high in carbohydrates. Unfortunately, these stimulate insulin production, which makes us hungry. Fats and proteins, on the other hand, are filling as well as sustaining. Fruit, salads, vegetables and whole grain bread are also rich in carbohydrates, and many of these foods contain a lot of sugar. A change in diet where you choose wisely which carbs to leave off, or at least to reduce, will cause you to eat less because you will be free of constant food cravings.

Rice contains starches, which are transformed to sugar relatively quickly. Here the term "carbohydrates" is synonymous with "sugar". According to the International Diabetes Federation, 72 million people in South-East Asia suffered from type 2 diabetes in 2013. In countries where rice is the staple food, this development is alarming. China has the highest diabetes rate worldwide, followed closely by India.

Our prescribed diet plan contained no rice whatsoever. Our new way of cooking, eating, and using familiar foods as well as incorporating new ones is very satisfying to this day. Constantly gaining more knowledge on the health benefits of certain foods and their effects on our systems never ceases to fascinate us. I couldn't get enough of researching and digging deeper as I went. We wondered why we had come upon all this information so late in our lives. What a shame! Why, for instance, hadn't any doctor ever told me that cinnamon lowers my blood sugar levels, and could be used, at the very least, to support my system suffering from type 2 diabetes? Or that amaranth helps with digestion and fights free radicals? That coconut oil and and quinoa can burn belly fat, and that coconut blossom nectar extract is a wonderful alternative to commonly used refined sugar? Etc, etc, etc. Why?

My hunger for knowledge was insatiable, and my sessions with Dr. K.S. got longer and longer. Soon I learned all about matcha tea, and how beneficial it was. And now I drink a cup of it at least once a day. Next, I found out about chia seeds and fell in love with them. While listening to valuable information on coconut oil - almost simultaneously - new insights on chlorophyll almost magically appeared. From chlorophyll, I graduated to phytonutrients, which in turn lead me to glutathione, and so on and so forth. It was all a revelation.

Not only had we entered a whole new world, we had also lost all those toxic, excess pounds, and our blood levels were now within the normal range, (please see page 212) leaving us happier and more content. I deeply regret having found all this valuable knowledge and having had all these phenomenal experiences so late in life. Which is why, dear reader, I truly wish for you to have this experience now, and for my work in this book to bring you great success.

Just imagine, looking at yourself in the mirror and seeing a slimmer, younger you - younger by five, ten or even fifteen years. And imagine further, how it will be, to suddenly feel a quantum leap in energy, and to find that when you get up in the morning, all your joint pains have vanished into thin air. All you have to do to make this come true, is follow through with the 7-day detox plan and then to make the reasonable adjustments to your diet which have been proven to be highly effective. After losing over 9 pounds with this wonderful detox plan in just a week, I, of course, had to tell all my girlfriends. Many of them asked me to send it to them. Out of many stories, I will tell you two. A dear colleague of mine, famous author Brigitte Riebe, wrote in an email, "Dear Katharina, this detox plan is phenomenal! Did you know that it stimulates your taste buds back to life? I had a potato today, and it tasted like a real potato! I haven't experienced that in such a long time." And Aveleen Avide, another writer colleague, reported having lost 8.3

pounds with this method, even though, on two evenings, she did not exactly follow the letter of the law. And just as remarkable was the fact that, in this short time, her waist narrowed by a more than an inch and a half!

I wrote this book to express my ongoing enthusiasm for our personal success and for having been blessed with this new way of eating. The truth is, that the evil, evil yo-yo effect never once made an appearance. I can honestly say: I. Am. Happy. I'm healthy, and most of all, deeply grateful. Maybe changing your diet or eating habits the way we did is more difficult for you - but you can, and will, find your way. And I can guarantee that changing to a new diet is the most effective way to lose weight, to regain and sustain good health. Because lasting fat reduction only occurs through selective and specific nutritional diet changes.

Scary Facts on Diabetes

According to the *German Health Report - Diabetes 2013*, approximately six million people in Germany were suffering from diabetes, 95 percent of whom had type 2 diabetes; 5 percent, meaning 300,000 people, had type 1 diabetes, among these, 30,000 were children and adolescents. The International Diabetes Federation reports that in 2013, worldwide, 387 million people were afflicted with the disease. The World Health Organization predicts a 50 (!) percent rise in connected fatalities by the year 2030. Diabetes has developed into a global epidemic, caused mainly by overweight, unhealthy diet, and lack of exercise. It is one of the root causes of blindness, amputation, and kidney failure. Diabetes is also responsible for premature death, brought about by cardio-vascular illnesses.

In 2013, 98 million people in China were registered as diabetics, and in all of South East Asia the total was 72 million. By 2030, this area is expected to register 123 million sufferers. 24 percent of Saudi-Arabia's population between the ages of twenty and seventy-nine were diagnosed with diabetes. Of all worldwide cases, type 2 diabetes constitutes 90 percent.

The number of children and teenagers, who, in the past, were more commonly afflicted by type 1 diabetes, due to genetic failure to produce sufficient insulin, has recently been increased by the addition of type 2 diabetics on a global scale. In some countries, almost half of all newly diagnosed cases are listed as type 2 diabetics. Type 2 diabetes can be prevented through healthy diet and sufficient exercise, whereas type 1 diabetes is heredity and cannot be cured.

On the Odyssey of Being a Woman

An odyssey is an adventurous voyage, taking the traveler from place to place, yet without necessarily leading directly to the sought-after destination. Most women find themselves on such a journey when it comes to losing weight. Because of "bad genes" sabotaging our every attempt to slim down, we are condemned to aimless wanderings much like on an odyssey. Losing fat is by far more challenging for women than it is for men because we are, in fact, not actually designed to be slim. I know this sounds grotesque, and even pretty mean, but it happens to be an irrefutable fact which becomes clear when we look back at our ancestors. Women's bodies are built specifically to store fat, which gives us energy and keeps us warm. Our female ancestors' job was to ensure survival and reproduction of the species, and fat - despite childbirth, milk production, and childrearing - was to be preserved at all costs. As opposed to today, women were not expected to look good. Unfortunately, from a genetic point of view, women are not at all capable of staying slim. Many factors make sure that our systems store fat. The most unfair fact is that our fat cells have far more and larger fat-storing enzymes than men. Their fat cells contain more and larger fat-burning enzymes than ours. *Damn!* And on top of it, our estrogen makes our fat cells multiply - almost like adding baking powder to a cake to make it rise. Consequently, we have fatty deposits on our rear ends, thighs and arms, which, much to our dismay, eventually turn into cellulite. And all this because it is in our genes to give birth, and we are called upon to ensure the survival of the species. So, girls, to make matters worse, by starving ourselves, we reduce our fat burning cells by a mere 50 percent. Hallelujah. Our bodies literally freak out and immediately flip the switch to fat-storing mode, which means that any crash diet creates the exact opposite of the desired results. Our fat burning enzymes are broken down, along with our muscle tissue, which actually help in the fat-burning process.

Men should please really listen to this: slim women almost always have to work much harder to get there. But then, we wouldn't want to jeopardize the survival of the species, would we? Especially since giving birth, watching the baby grow up and feeling its love is a wonderful experience. And still, we want to be slim and beautiful. So how are we supposed to manage this impossible balancing act?

The Liver's Role in Weight Loss

The key player in weight loss is our liver, also known as "the chemical factory", Dr. K.S. explained to me in great detail. Among other important tasks, our liver eliminates toxins from our system and also secretes bile, or digestive fluid, to break down fats in our small intestine. The bile produced by the liver is extremely important for the digestion of fats. When our stomach is empty, bile is intermediately stored in the gall bladder. We can survive without our gallbladder, should it need removing due to gallstones. However, some people have trouble digesting fatty foods after the removal. A balanced diet with lots of fibers along with regular exercising is best for them. Furthermore, consuming fatty foods on a regular basis is not a good idea. Yet, not only too much food, but too little can also be harmful. Unhealthy eating, fasting and certain diets can cause damage by disrupting the balance of gall bladder fluids. A dysfunctional liver can also cause problems in cholesterol suppression. In our Western culture, we are prone to consuming cholesterol-rich foods and that leads directly to weight problems. When our liver has trouble metabolizing fat, we gain weight - mainly in our abdominal region. Our bellies protrude, and we have a so-called beer-belly, or paunch. The extra fatty tissue below the upper abdomen, also known as love handles, are a further sign of liver dysfunction. Its ability to filter out the abundant fat particles in our bloodstream has been compromised, causing them to accumulate elsewhere, for example, in the form of fatty deposits under our skin. Enter dreaded cellulite, which goes straight to our thighs, bottom, arms and belly. Getting rid of those fat deposits is very difficult if liver function is not restored. This is another reason why we gain weight and lose our shape with age. When our liver is overwhelmed and full of garbage, so to speak, we're not able to lose weight adequately, no matter how many diets or how much exercise we subject ourselves to. This also explains the yo-yo effect. The phenomenon of regaining lost fat, immediately following a diet, is a consequence of liver dysfunction. For us, as women, in order to juggle the survival of the species and staying slim, we need our liver to function properly. With Dr. K.S'. detox plan, women and men alike are able to support and cleanse their liver, giving their metabolism a jump start, around the clock, even while asleep. While certain toxins are flushed out with bile fluids, others are made water soluble to be eliminated with urine through the kidneys.

Tips for Liver Support by Dr. K.S.

- Every day, take a tablespoon of liquid cold-pressed coconut oil before every meal.
- Eat mostly fresh foods.
- Drink up to 6 pints of non-refrigerated non-carbonated water during the day, every day.
- Incorporate lots of fiber and whole grain foods in your daily diet.
- Eat artichokes. They stimulate bile production.
- Supplement with vitamin C and calcium to support lead elimination.
- Supplement with selenium and zinc to further mercury elimination (found, for instance, in amalgam dental fillings).
- Take a daily dose of milk thistle, in capsule form. It strengthens, protects and regenerates the liver.
- Treat yourself to lymphatic drainage, foot reflex zone and connective tissue massages, as well as sauna-baths and dry-brushing of your skin.
- Cut down your sugar intake.
- Avoid refined white flour and all milk products and reduce your animal protein consumption.

Exercise – Sorry, Not My Favorite

Winston Churchill once famously said: "No sports, just whiskey and cigars!" Let me just leave it at "no sports". Because, of course, I understand that sports and exercise not only help us burn calories, but is also good for our digestion, mobility, and helps us lose weight, to mention only a few of their benefits. "Exercising ensures a longer life", says the Department for Public Health and Caring Sciences of Uppsala, Sweden. Exercise prevents obesity and consequent illnesses. My better half exercises for an hour, three times a week. And it shows. I envy him. If there were a pill which provided the same benefits as sports and exercise, with no side-effects, I'd be the first to take it - even though, just thirty minutes of bicycling or jogging, three times a week, would be enough to reduce the risk of osteoporosis by one third, according to a study by the German Sport University of Cologne. One look at our ancestors clearly shows us why moving is essential to us even to this very day. To secure their survival, the stone-age hunters had to cover great distances - researchers say over 24 miles a day. Since physical demands have not changed significantly in millennia, even I, with a strong aversion to exercise, understand the down side of a sedentary life-style. To activate and boost our metabolism, we need to move. That's just the way it is! What really pleased me, was to find that daily activities also burn calories.

Even lying down, we use up an average of 68 calories, just sitting, approximately 70 calories, and walking at 2.2 miles an hour burns 210 calories per hour. Of course that isn't much to write home about, but it's better than nothing!

So, you can easily do better than I. Move, as much as you personally can, every day! And your gut will thank you.

Nature's Superfoods

In the following chapters I have compiled everything I found useful to help me follow through with changing my diet. I do not claim that my research is perfect, yet I carried it out with great care and diligence, and am thoroughly convinced I have done the right thing. I am aware that there will always be people with more knowledge than I, and that new research is constantly updating current findings. Nor am I revealing any sensational secrets of eternal youth. Or am I? Be that as it may, in just ten months, Dr. K.S. made it possible for us once again to enjoy our lives to the fullest once again. We feel greatly indebted to him. We're bursting with health and vitality, and my approval rating of him has sky-rocketed, despite his tendency to ramble on. Truth be told, he is kind of a chatterbox. But then again, he taught me so many things I would never have known. In the wise words of the Dalai Lama: "When you speak you are only repeating what you know; but when you listen, you may actually learn something new." Which once again goes to show, that there are - and should be - two ways of looking at things. In the meantime, we became devout amaranth and quinoa eaters. We switched the piles of plastic containers in our kitchen for glass, we cook exclusively with coconut oil, spice our meals with rock or pink Himalayan (crystal) salt.

We love matcha tea and chia seeds, we make our own "milk", our own coconut oil, bake our own bread and supplement our diet with the miraculous papain enzymes and much, much more. Please do not think I have reinvented the wheel and turned into the all-knowing health and slimness queen or anti-ageing goddess. Everything in this book is known and well-established. It is based on many conversations with Dr. K.S., the research found in conventional as well as alternative medical literature, and our personal rich experience with cooking and eating new foods.

The Coconut: A True Globetrotter

The globetrotting coconut is loved worldwide. If it falls in the sea, the fruit can float for long distances and still germinate to form new trees after being washed ashore. There are stories of still viable coconuts that made it all the way to Scandinavia. Humans have cultivated the coconut palm for over 3000 years. Besides the fruit, the leaves and trunk are still used today to make brooms, furniture, and even huts and boats. For millions of people, the coconut is a staple food. It provides everything needed for survival. There are hundreds of reports of castaways surviving for months on little more than coconuts. Here in Malaysia, it is customary to smash a coconut at the doorstep to bring wealth and good fortune.

The Malaysians make a wonderful delicacy, called "kaya", out of the fruit, which is a sweet, caramel-colored spread - a kind of coconut jam. The name "kaya" means rich, and that it is - rich in calories - and everybody loves it. This overwhelmingly delicious and exotic treat is very popular in all of Malaysia as well as in neighboring Singapore. Beware: while enjoying this smooth, silky coconut jam on a piece of warm crispy toast, along with a cup of "kopi", meaning coffee, there is a serious risk of addiction.

"Kaya" is made of eggs, coconut milk, coconut blossom sugar and the aromatic pandan leaf. The mere mention of "kaya" evokes childhood memories in most Malaysians, of standing in the kitchen with their mothers and grandmothers, watching them prepare the delightful jam. The ingredients are carefully beaten with the traditional whisk in a cauldron suspended above an open charcoal fire, until they turn golden brown and become silky in texture. Kaya comes in various shades of yellow, green or brown. Some prefer a thinner consistency, while others prefer the thicker version. The traditional method requires stirring the jelly for hours in a double-boiler, whereas today, a simple bain-marie will do the trick. With modern kitchen appliances, in as little as thirty minutes, you can easily create a jam just as satiny and smooth as in old times. (see page 247).

Coconut Water - Not Just a Trendy Drink

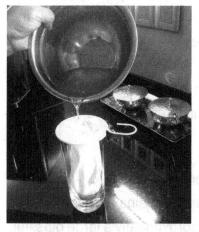

Even though opening the coconut may be challenging for Europeans, inside there a precious treasure, coconut water. Not to be confused with canned or boxed coconut milk, this fluid is clear, full of wonderful nutrients and low in calories. Mango and other tropical fruit store a great deal of water, but only the coconut can deliver 8 oz. in a shell.

Natural coconut water contains inorganic ions such as copper, zinc, and manganese and similar amounts of salts and nutrients found in our blood. In an emergency on the Pacific front in World War Two, it was used as a replacement for plasma.

Because the coconut's husk completely seals in a one hundred percent sterile fluid, people living here in these tropical regions use it to clean wounds, and even for rehydration in severe cases of diarrhea. The National Institute of Health states that the nutrient's composition does not quite meet the recommended norms required to restore the body's water balance. However, in the middle of the jungle, coconut water is often the only help available.

An excellent thirst quencher, coconut water is far better than any soft drink, especially in this tropical climate. It doesn't burden our system, is low in fat and sugar, and is loaded with healthy ingredients especially popular with athletes. The widespread coconut water products now found, even on the European market, come nowhere near the pure fresh coconut water of a young green fruit.

Nutrients Contained in Coconut Water
The hermetically sealed husk contains an average of 8 ounces of coconut water - approximately a large glassful. This most valuable, nutrient rich fluid comes from the young green nut. It contains trace elements such as iron, iodine, copper, manganese, and zinc. Minerals found in it are calcium, potassium, magnesium, sodium and phosphorus, as well as vitamins B1, B2, B3, B5, B6 and B9, folic acid, and vitamin C. One large glass of coconut water covers 35 percent of our daily requirement of potassium (700 mg), 25 percent of magnesium (75 mg), 7 percent of calcium (67.5 mg), 21 percent of sodium (117.5 mg) and 10 percent of phosphorus (75 mg). Coconut water contains about 0.58 gr. of salt, 1 gr. fat, 0.87 unsaturated fats, and only 12 gr. of sugar.

BY THE WAY: In 2003, we took our daughter on a short beach trip to Penang - a wonderfully beautiful place to visit, full of interesting and mysterious traditions - when our daughter suddenly broke out with a rash from sun allergy. A waiter rushed to bring us a fresh coconut, saying: "She should drink the water, better yet, the water of two coconuts, that'll help." And lo and behold, shortly after downing two coconut water drinks, the allergy vanished.

Coconut Oil: A Modern Day Medicine

Dr. K.S. firmly insisted that from now on, we exclusively use coconut oil for cooking, and especially for frying. He had already mentioned that this oil could burn belly fat, but it is able to do much, much more.

When ingested, the topical oil extracted from the coconut flesh acts as a sort of blast furnace, kick starting our metabolism and burning fat, especially visceral fats in the abdominal area. These fats are by no means harmless because they hide deep down in our abdominal cavity and collect around our organs. They're particularly insidious because they produce inflammatory proteins, hormones, and fatty acids, thereby impairing proper functioning of our vital organs. They are regarded as one of the main causes of serious diseases connected to obesity, such as heart attack, stroke, and diabetes. And worst of all, these dangerous fatty deposits are not outwardly visible. They can also easily get inflamed, adding to the risk factors. Via the portal vein, inflammatory factors flow directly to the liver and consequently flood our entire system. The portal vein is the connection between two capillary systems. Its task is to collect the blood from our abdominal organs - the stomach, intestines, pancreas and spleen - and to carry it directly to the liver.

When our cells are under constant inflammatory attack, they eventually become resistant to insulin, and we develop type 2 diabetes. If, in addition, our arteries get inflamed, a stroke or a heart attack becomes a real possibility. The widely underestimated danger lurking in our insides is caused by the visceral fat cell's highly active metabolism. Coconut oil is able to break down these dangerous fats and enhance weight loss.

Every day, before breakfast and dinner, and sometimes even in between, we take a tablespoon of coconut oil.

Worldwide, the healthiest people are those with a diet rich in coconut. In the thirties, Dr. Weston Price found that South Pacific Islanders had no concept of heart disease whatsoever. In 1981, two researchers encountered the same phenomenon in a Polynesian community which also subsisted mainly on coconuts. They found the inhabitants to be fit and in excellent cardio-vascular health. Where were all the blocked arteries and heart attacks, despite the large quantities of "evil" unsaturated fats in their diet? Clearly, the coconuts had done no harm to their hearts. The coconut's health benefits are, and have always been, well-known to the inhabitants of tropical countries. Koh Samui, an island in the Gulf of Thailand, has the coconut as its emblem. Thailand exports over two million coconuts per month! Thai coconuts are believed to be the best in the world, containing the "kopra", derived from its core.

I remember that my mother always used coconut fat. Later, margarine and butter became more fashionable for cooking and baking. Today, we know more about the hazards of margarine, which we jokingly like to call "plastic butter". In the following pages, you will find out more about what cholesterol suppressing margarine really does to our systems.

Coconut oil is rich in fatty acids - lauric acid being an especially valuable one, with its ability to fight viruses, bacteria and parasites. Interestingly, caprylic acid, another fatty acid contained in coconuts, has now been put on the list of antimicrobial ingredients in coconuts. Coconut oil's use is now FDA approved to be reinstated in kitchens, bakeries and fast-food restaurants. Coconut oil is highly heat resistant and doesn't turn into harmful trans fats during the cooking process.

The food industry is well aware that the healthy properties found in the oil make it far superior to commonly sold cooking oils. Increasingly, recent scientific studies show that lauric and caprylic acids are getting more respect. For four decades now, the benefits of coconut fatty acids have been well known to a select group of researchers, laying the groundwork for twenty further research papers and numerous American patents. Leading scientist in the field is Mary G. Enig. In her article "Coconut: In Support of Good Health in the 21st Century", she describes the anti-micro-bacterial advantages of coconut oil.

To reiterate, the good reasons for the daily use and consumption of coconut oil are: it helps prevent, reduce, and fight viruses, fungus, and bacteria. It lowers high blood pressure, fights colds, allergies, psoriasis, herpes, venereal disease, and free radicals. It keeps teeth and gums healthy, supports prostate health, and enhances weight loss. When taken before meals, a tablespoon of coconut oil lessens your appetite and helps regulate the balance of good HDL cholesterol and bad LDL cholesterol. Studies also show that the system does not convert coconut oil to body fat as easily as other cooking fats, and thereby the risk of cardio-vascular disease, heart-attack, and stroke is decreased.

Coconut Oil for a Healthy Brain

The fatty acids contained in coconut oil boost the body's ketone production. Our organs and tissues function better when supplied with ketone as a fuel and energy source. Since the same applies to the brain and the heart, obviously brain function in healthy people as well as Alzheimer patients can be improved with coconut oil. Scientists found Alzheimer patients to be suffering from deficient brain energy, which led to the development of a drug called "Axona", which boosts ketone production.

Dr. Mary T. Newport, medical director of the New-Born Intensive-Care Unit at Spring Hill Regional Hospital heard about this medication when her husband started showing the initial symptoms of the disease in 2003.

She began studying scientific findings and soon decided that, instead of giving her husband the drug, to give him coconut oil instead. After many years of medication and the ensuing side effects, Steve's condition had deteriorated. He could not remember how to draw the face of a clock, nor did he know what day it was. Dr. Mary Newport started by giving him two teaspoons of coconut oil per day, soon increasing the dose to several tablespoons and adding it to his food. Steve's condition improved rapidly, until he could finally remember the date and was able to draw the face of a clock again. "It was as if the oil had flipped a switch in his brain, enabling him to think more clearly again", Mary later said. The 37-day coconut therapy further allowed Steve to perfect his clock drawing. After another five months, the patient's vision problems cleared up to the point of being able to take up reading again, and the tremors he suffered from lessened considerably. His interest in the people around him was rekindled. Mary carried on with her tireless research on the effects of coconut oil on Alzheimer's and published the wonderful news of her husband's remarkable progress. She even started a blog on her experiences with the disease.

Coconut Oil in the Bathroom and Kitchen

In tropical countries coconut oil is not only a common food but is also used as an effective hair and skin care product. It prevents hair damage and works as a skin moisturizer. It may not be coincidental that the people who eat a lot of coconut and use its oil for skin care have especially nice skin, shiny hair and a certain glow. You can apply it to dry skin, massage it into towel dry hair, you can even use it as a make-up remover. Just be careful not to get it in your eyes. It won't cause any damage, but will leave an unpleasant oil film on your eye. Experts now assume that lauric acid strengthens the immune systems of newborns and grown-ups alike. Lauric acid contained in coconut oil is also found in breast milk. Numerous other beneficial properties are attributed to lauric acid such as improved absorption of calcium, magnesium, and all soluble vitamins (A, D, E and K) and, as mentioned earlier, it gives a general metabolic boost.

The delicate coconut taste adds a fine note to any dish, without being overpowering. Because cold pressed coconut oil is not heated during the production process, all natural ingredients are preserved. I use it when frying fish, meat and vegetables, in salad dressings, cake and home-made power bars, and I even make my own ice cream, candy, and chocolates with this delicious oil. We also use it as a body lotion and as a replacement for commercial deodorant (see also page 229).

Evaluating Quality Coconut Oil

To obtain extremely high quality coconut oil, the following production criteria are vital: upon opening the nut, the flesh of the fruit must be pressed immediately. The contained milk is centrifuged, leaving concentrated coconut fat, which is then cooled down to minus 4 degrees Fahrenheit. This procedure extracts remaining water in the fat. Next, the fat is melted down at 104 degrees Fahrenheit and again centrifuged to extract the very last of any water remaining. To obtain clear coconut oil, it must be filtered through cellulose filters repeatedly until it is crystal clear. Be sure to ask your retailer how his coconut oil is produced.

Be aware that when stored below 77 degrees Fahrenheit room temperature, the oil will begin to solidify and take on a whitish color. This has no bearing on the quality. Currently, in Germany, the selection of coconut oil is not all that diverse. Finding liquid oil in bottles is almost impossible. Various distributors offer coconut oil in small glass containers, but only in solid, white form. Recognizing good quality oil is important. In any case, it should be cold pressed. The good news is, you can also make your own coconut oil (see page 232).

If you find cooking with coconut oil too expensive, there are other ways to use it to support your health. Before breakfast every day, take a tablespoon of coconut oil and gargle with it for ten minutes, before spitting it out. Then, brush your teeth.

Or, just before breakfast, take or drink a tablespoon of the oil. Dr. K.S. recommends the following doses according to body weight:

* up to 22 lbs: 1 Tbsp.
* up to 44.1 lbs: 1½ Tbsp.
* up to 66.1 lbs: 2 Tbsp.
* up to 88.2 lbs: 2½ Tbsp.
* up to 110.2 lbs: 3 Tbsp.
* up to 132.2 lbs: 3½ Tbsp.
* up to 154.3 lbs: 4 Tbsp.
* over 154 lbs: 5 Tbsp.

Don't worry about taking too much, because with coconut oil, "more helps more". Thanks to its immunity stimulating and anti-micro bacterial effect, an over-dose is highly unlikely. Coconut oil is a superfood and not a medicine.

The Many Uses of Coconut Oil

One day, I bought some locally produced coconut oil on Koh Samui Island. Its taste was not quite as refined as that of our homemade version, but in the packaging I found a brochure with an interesting statement which I would like to quote here: "Coconut oil is a functional food. It is not a medicine, it is a food of modern medicine." Below you will find an overview of uses.

* for pan and deep-frying, baking and cooking
* as a substitute for butter

* as a supplement for daily energy
* for dry cuticles
* as a make-up remover
* for the prevention of stretch marks
* to support healthy thyroid function
* for removal of newborn cradle cap: apply massaging gently, wait and carefully swab with a lukewarm washcloth
* mixed with apple vinegar, to get rid of lice
* mixed with rock or pink Himalaya salt, as a foot skin scrub
* mixed with sugar, as a body scrub in the shower
* applied on dry skin areas, for moisture on lips, elbows, feet etc.
* as a hair conditioner for dry hair and split ends treatment: leave in dry hair under shower cap for several hours, wash and rinse thoroughly
* as an fungus preventative
* alleviates allergy symptoms when massaged into nasal mucous membranes
* destroys intestinal parasites and yeast overgrowth
* enhances healthy gum tissue
* can substitute other vegetable oils in any recipe
* relieves painful sunburns
* as a natural lubricant in the case of vaginal flora imbalance
* as an anti-bacterial skin lotion (also for acne)
* as an after-shave lotion

* relieves itchiness in mosquito bites and chicken pox
* alleviates hemorrhoid pains: apply externally
* when rubbed gently in to damp hair tips, adds moisture and softness
* coconut oil compresses for dry skin areas: drench gauze or linen cloth in liquid oil, place on dry area for several hours. To avoid spots, cellophane wrap compress
* add to warm water foot bath: softens hardened areas and is a fungus preventative
* spread thinly as a body lotion. Fast absorption, but wait 10 to 15 minutes before putting clothes on!
* a reliable deodorant for several hours: after showering, apply directly to armpits
* a tablespoon in your bathwater makes your skin smooth and silky
* for baby's diaper rash, apply on irritated areas
* for breast-feeding moms, take 3 to 4 tablespoons daily to stimulate milk production and add nutrients
* apply to tender nipples, coconut oil is soothing

Important to Know

Since the end of the 19th century in Germany, a fat used for baking and frying called "Palmin" could be found in almost every kitchen. We wondered about this staple product because on the package it says, "made of 100 percent coconut fat". But taking a closer look and comparing the low price of Palmin with that of cold pressed coconut oil, we had serious doubts. In any case, Palmin is by no means an organic virgin product, and whether or not it is chemically processed remains highly controversial. According to the manufacturers, it contains only 0.1 percent trans fats and only air is pumped into the mass, to provide a texture optimal for cutting into pieces. Not even "Palmin Soft" is allowed in our fridge. The label indicates that it consists mainly of sunflower oil, palm oil, palm kernel fat and one part coconut fat. As a general rule, trans fats appear on the labeling as "hardened fats", "hardened vegetable oils" or "partly hardened vegetable oils". Also to be avoided are refined oils and fats. Here the base product, such as the coconut fruit flesh (copra), is heated and chemically treated to extract the oil. In the process, it loses its original color, its taste, and is sold as "neutral in flavor". Lastly, it is put through another elaborate cleansing process, in other words, refined. Be sure to avoid these products at all cost. For us, pure, cold pressed, native coconut oil is the only way to go.

INCIDENTALLY: Even if many chefs fry food in cold pressed olive oil, please do not! At high temperatures, olive oil turns into dangerous and harmful trans fats. Unfortunately, many TV Chefs not only recommend it, but actually use it themselves. I addressed this with famous TV and star-chef Alfred Schuhbeck, who agreed with me and highly praised the virtues of coconut oil.

If you don't like coconut oil or can't stand the taste of it, you can use ghee as a perfect alternative. Ghee is cleared butter which has been used in Ayurvedic cuisine and medicine for centuries. In the early 80's in India, ghee and coconut oil were accused of being responsible for high cholesterol, causing many people to switch to other, supposedly cholesterol-free, plant oils. Yet, eventually, India saw its error, realizing it could no longer gloss over the significant increase in diabetes and cardio-vascular disease. Since then, ghee and coconut oil have been readmitted into Indian cuisine. Our body processes the medium-chain fatty acids (MCT) contained in coconut oil much the same way it does carbohydrates, primarily to obtain energy quickly. Because medium-chain fatty acids stimulate the metabolism more than proteins do, and do not require bile to be digested, they are the ideal fats for athletes. Even with impaired fat digestion issues, coconut oil is well assimilated.

Gula Malacca: The Sweet Blossom

Besides its fruit flesh, oil and water, the coconut harbors another very special treasure, the sap from its flower bud, out of which, for centuries, coconut sugar has been rendered by hand. A cut is made in the flower bud, and the sap begins to flow from it. For this, the farmer has to climb to the top of the coconut palm to hang up hollow bamboo stems and collect the sap. The interesting thing about this is, that once the cut is made, the sap will then flow for the next seventy (!) years. This means that a farmer who plants a palm as a child, will be able to harvest it for a life time. This allows plantations to be sustainable and protects the environment against tropical deforestation. It is important to begin the sugar manufacturing as quickly as possible after harvesting to avoid fermentation. Industrial production is hardly possible, since the sap cannot survive lengthy transportation.

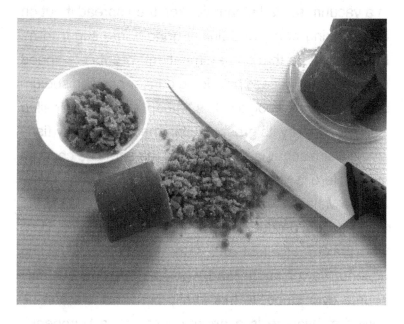

Unfermented sap is essential to the production of pure tropical, unrefined sugar. Next, the sap is filtered to remove any impurities. Since strength lies within serenity, the next phase of the process is executed with great calm and patience. As it is traditionally customary, the sweet mass is now placed over an open wood fire until it transforms into a syrupy substance, along with a small piece of coconut placed in the pot, to keep it from boiling over. Smart tip: the same works for pasta water. The syrup is then placed in a big wok to let it thicken further, until it reaches its unique malt and caramel-like taste. To cool off, the hot syrup is poured into bamboo containers, giving it its classical cylindrical shape.

Modern manufacturers reduce the crystallized mass in a vacuum sealed steam cooker, then spread it out on large baking pans, and finally grind it into sugar form. Please beware that some "impatient" producers speed up the drying process by adding cancer-causing sodium sulfite! You can recognize this "cheap" sugar, often called "palm sugar", by its greenish shimmer and slightly fishy smell. Palm sugar is by no means the same as coconut sugar! Here in Malaysia, the real thing goes by the name of Gula Malacca and is sold everywhere. Fortunately, we found a local producer right in his own huge plantation, who makes excellent and extremely delicious tasting coconut flower sugar, and who has become our only source ever since. In this family business, we can be sure that hygiene is a priority, just as we Europeans have come to expect it.

An Exotic Sugar Conquers the World

For centuries now, coconut sugar has been a staple food in South-East Asian culture. In 2010, it was voted one of the top ten trendy health foods by People Magazine - and for good reason. Not only is it an authentic natural product, but is also a much healthier alternative to ordinary sweeteners. It can replace white sugar, brown, and cane sugar, agave and other types of syrup. It may sound like it tastes of coconut, however it tastes completely different. Its characteristic caramel flavor literally melts in your mouth, and ends on a delicate and surprisingly malty note. Its low melting point allows it to dissolve quickly, whether in cold or in hot fluids. I have even come to use it instead of honey, in one of my own creations, with pandan leaves (Pandan leaves are commonly used as a flavor in South-East Asian cuisine).

Coconut sugar has countless properties not only relevant in the kitchen. For example, its low glycemic index (GI), compared with the dextrose GI of 100, lies at no more than 35; meaning that its assimilation by the blood is slower than that of ordinary sugars. Analysis found it abundant in nutrients - among them magnesium, iron, calcium, zinc, vitamins B1, B3, B6 and C, which are very uncommon in sugars.

For cooking and baking, it works exactly the same way as normal sugar. In tropical cuisine, the crystallized blossom nectar is often used to flavor meats, fish and fried dishes. It gives Peking Duck skin a nice gloss. In various desserts, like Mimpi Manis, it is a must and a wonderful, sweet seduction. Recently, this exotic sugar made quite a name for itself in New York with "Pumpkin-Spice-Latte", made with coconut flower sugar. It was a total hit (see recipe page 253).

The Tropical Miracle Fruit: Papaya

"Evolution most likely places the cradle of humanity in tropical regions, maybe in Africa", Dr. K.S. declared one day, and I knew he was getting ready for another long lecture. "Which could mean that we may have a genetic adaptation to exotic fruit, like mango, papaya and pineapple", I quickly interrupted, because I sensed where he was going with this. His assumption was based on an astonishing reflex observed in newborns. An apple placed directly under a baby's nose causes no reaction whatsoever, whereas a mango under its nose triggers an immediate sucking reflex.

Tropical fruit is much richer in nutrients and enzymes than fruit types found in western latitudes. Enzymes play an important role for humans, but also for the fruit itself, especially for the papaya. As opposed to most tropical fruit with a hard shell for protection against insects and other insurgents, papayas have a regular killer-enzyme to protect them from within. And this very special enzyme is papain.

Bye-Bye, Cellulite!

Here' the great news for anyone wanting to be slim: the papaya enzyme, papain - and this is my own true, personal experience - has the ability to melt away fatty deposits! It is able to break down proteins, very much like pancreatic enzymes, which stimulate digestion, and prevent fat deposits. After Dr. K.S.'s promising two hour discourse on papain - which I have a lot more to say about - I started taking a daily dose of papain, two capsules, three times a day, over a period of six months, feeling skeptical yet full of expectations. Then one sunny day, slim as I was now, I dared try on a new bathing suit and was just taking a last scrutinizing glance to be sure, when I could not believe what I saw. Breasts, belly and legs. *Hello? Thighs? What happened to my cellulite???* Incredulously, I touched my skin. *Completely smooth! This is impossible.*

I was on cloud nine. This was beyond all expectation. It felt like lightening had struck, as though the German National Lottery had told me I'd hit the multi-million Euro jack-pot. My cellulite never really caused me major distress - it was just the way it was. This minor beauty issue wasn't the worst of my worries. It was far more important to me to regain my health and to become slim enough to wear pretty new clothes again, without having to hide under layers of clothing.

I believe that the papain enzyme, with its reputation for efficiency, did an impressive and amazing job.

Wow, right!? You must be wondering how this works.

Papain not only breaks down proteins, but is also able to detoxify the system, ridding it of unwelcome waste substances. These are clogging our system due to poor diet and lack of exercise, thus slowing down our natural metabolism.

An interesting fact: in tropical regions, meat is wrapped in papaya leaves over night to tenderize it, while in Central and South America, papaya has been used as a health remedy for centuries. In Hawaii people say, "A papaya a day, keeps the doctor away." And rightly so! Its abundance in valuable enzymes can hardly be beaten. And researchers have been well aware of its "magic powers" for some time now. Also, papaya contains no fruit acid whatsoever, making it suitable for diabetics. And that is by no means all. But one step at a time. By the end of the 20th century, from the unripe fruit and leaves, scientists were able to isolate the highly effective papain enzyme contained mainly in its seeds but also in its outer skin. This so-called proteolytic enzyme is one of several digestive enzymes capable of breaking down protein chains for better assimilation. It does not, however, break down fats, as is often mentioned erroneously. In our system, there are approximately 30 billion biochemical reactions occurring per second, every single one induced by enzymes. Our bodies harbor an estimated 10,000 different enzymes, only 2,000 of which have been scientifically researched and recorded.

The Many Things One Enzyme Can Do

All the beneficial ingredients contained in this "health bomb" sustain a perfect balance and are found in all parts of the plant. They're in the roots, the stem, in the leaves and flowers, the skin, the flesh, the milk and even in the seeds. This means that nearly every part of the plant is usable for medicinal purposes. The green papaya contains 5,000 percent (!) more papain and has greater healing power than when it is ripe. Here is an overview of some of the wonderful properties papain has to offer:

* The highly potent papaya enzymes attack only diseased tissue, which can develop into cancer, while healthy cells are left intact. The reason for this is the protective mechanism they have to ward off voracious, protein catabolism. Cancer cells however, are slow and able to produce protective substances only after 12 to 48 hours.
* Papain is used as a preventative for cardio-vascular disease like heart attack and stroke by breaking down fibrin and fibrinogen. These two substances are responsible for blood clotting that can lead to serious health problems.
* For premenopausal women, papain is very effective for balancing the menstrual cycle, mood swings, and fatigue. It curtails excessive chin hair growth, hair loss, and bloating. It slows the ageing process of cells, and ensures sounder sleep.

* Scientists have even found the papaya fruit to have antibacterial, anti-inflammatory and antioxidant properties.
* Papain helps digest gliadin, a component in gluten, thereby reducing, and in some cases, even removing gluten intolerance altogether. This makes the enzyme highly valuable to people with gluten intolerance.

Papaya's Anti-Aging Properties

According to ancient Chinese wisdom, "Papaya is the fruit of long-life". In the 15th century, Portuguese navigator, Vasco da Gama, praised the papaya for its rejuvenating properties and called it the "Tree of Eternal Youth".

Modern man, rushing from one appointment to the next, has long been searching for an effective way to counter stress. As menopause is difficult for women, all forms of stress contribute to the ageing process. The enzyme papain turns out to be an important balancing factor. 77 percent of menopausal women, aged over 47, participating in a study on papain, stated that their symptoms were significantly "alleviated" and in some cases "barely noticeable". I can certainly say the same for myself.

*Dr. B. Lytton Benard, of The Health Centre in Guadalajara, does not limit papaya's cleansing effect to the digestive system, but contends it affects all other tissue as well. "The key to rejuvenation and longevity in full possession of our powers, lies within the papaya". Dr. Norman W. Walker, since 1910, New York head of Norwalk-Laboratorium for Nutrition and Science, confirms the rejuvenating effect, after decades of research and papers on healthy living and longevity. As far back as the 'thirties he said: "Nature has given us everything we need to stay healthy from cradle to grave. It doesn't take that much. The greatest gift of all is natural food. The secret to a fulfilled and long life lies in a healthy diet. It is not really a secret!" Walker explained the papaya was instrumental in rejuvenation by stimulating and harmonizing our glandular system.

Dr. K.S. attributes these effects to the increased release of HGH hormones, known in medical terms as the "human-growth-hormone". It is produced by the pituitary gland (hypophysis), and is one of the most important regulatory hormones in our system. It influences virtually all functions. Our whole life, HGH controls cell renewal and liver regeneration, bone density, brain function, and enzyme production. It further ensures healthy skin, muscle tissue and cartilage, as well as strong and pretty nails. It rejuvenates our heart, liver, and kidneys, revitalizes our immune system, and improves our sexual and emotional functions. The intake of papain causes the production of arginine, the amino acid which then prompts the pituitary gland to secrete more HGH, thus achieving the rejuvenation effect. HGH controls cell deterioration and protects our tissue from tumors and cancer. Because enzymes keep our glandular and our entire system young, and because with age our enzyme production increasingly diminishes, an effective way to slow the ageing process is the regular intake of enzyme-rich papaya and pineapple.

How Papain Supports the Immune System

In the presence of internationally renowned scientists presenting papers on papaya, French Nobel Prize laureate and virologist Professor Luc Montagnier was called upon to defend the effectiveness of papain. He found that when added to the Triple Drug Therapy for AIDS patients, it accelerated immune system reconstruction demonstrably. Montagnier proved thereby that the body is able to "heal itself", regardless of the type of disease in question. To "achieve this miracle", it is necessary to provide a helping hand to the regenerative system by administering ample antioxidants. Voilà! And that is exactly what papain has to offer. As a reminder, Montagnier clearly praised its antioxidant properties.

The papaya enzyme's ability to eliminate intestinal worms such as tapeworms, roundworms and maggots, are especially appreciated in tropical countries. Children are particularly susceptible to these because of their tendency to frequently put their fingers in their mouths. In Indonesia, papaya serves as a malaria preventative. And although many regions there are considered malaria-free, there are sufficient areas with serious problems. The local population has a multitude of traditional remedies for malaria, one of them a tea made of papaya leaves. Foreign aid workers experienced similar positive results with it in other tropical countries. But please beware! The use of papaya leaves is NOT to be mistaken for an anti-malaria drug! If you have malaria symptoms, you must immediately consult a doctor. There are no verified scientific studies on malaria prevention with papaya .

On the other hand, papaya is incredibly useful in fighting stress. Stress affecting the elderly is especially high in urban environments. As a petri dish for obscure bacterial cultures, city water pipes, for example, largely contribute to an increase in toxicity and ageing - not to mention obesity, and smoking and alcohol abuse in the last fifty years. Women with a history of employment and those still working, and aged between 38 and 65, are particularly affected by environmental pollution and stress. Studies on working women show that this target group has great need for wellbeing and seeks strategies for stress reduction.

A group of 18 healthy men, aged from 20 to 35, took part in a random blind study. Its objective was to determine the effect of papain on various biochemical parameters and the immune system in a situation similar to that of flying. The study was standardized for military personnel, pilots and astronauts, and professionals exposed to a hostile working environment. Before going to sleep, and prior to a physically strenuous event or stressful situation due to flight simulation, subjects were given fermented papaya fruit. The results suggest that fermented papaya acts as an anti-stress agent, helping our system to adapt to the stress caused by lack of oxygen, physical over-straining, or psycho-emotional factors.

Papaya's Antioxidant Effects

Our bodies are made up of an estimated 100 billion cells, 20 billion of which are brain cells. That is not counting approximately the same number of bacteria and other single or multi-celled organisms colonizing our bodies. Fifty million cells die in our system per second. But not to worry, just as many new ones replace them. Simultaneously however, our cells are attacked up to 10,000 times by free radicals on a daily basis.

The consequence is cell destruction. Many diseases, along with premature ageing, are the result of cell deterioration caused by free radicals.

While, in fact, free radicals in themselves, are not really all that dangerous. It's actually the imbalance between free radicals and antioxidants that poses the real danger. This is very common in most people today. Free radicals are not all bad though, because they attack not only healthy cells but the sick ones as well, making them harmless.

Free radicals are not merely a by-product of our cell's oxygen exchange. Excessive alcohol consumption, stress, excessive sun-bathing, smoking and toxic environmental and nutritional substances all stimulate free radical production. Many of us experience stress in the work place. And even on vacation, when we're finally about to recover from all the work related stress and enjoy the sunshine, we find ourselves at the mercy of free radical attacks.

"What actually happens, when free radicals assault our bodies?", I was asking Dr. K.S., although I was fully aware that his answer would not be a short one. "They're oxygen particles which are belligerent, so to speak", he began, "with only a single electron. This drives them to go in search of another electron, causing a devastating chain reaction. When they find a particle with two electrons, they steal one out of the other's pair, breaking up its electron couple and the chain reaction is launched. And because the "robbed" oxygen particle is now also left with half an electron pair, it too, goes in search of its "missing" part. And the little buggers aren't choosy either. Any old particle will do."

Papaya is able to help ward off this destruction with the help of its antioxidant cell protector vitamins, which are vitamin C and carotene. Papaya is higher in vitamin C than oranges and kiwis and contains more carotene than carrots.

BY THE WAY: At the time, for about a year, I had been feeling listless, was suffering from hot flashes, depression, nervousness and sudden outbreaks of sweat. I started taking two papain capsules, three times a day after meals, and gradually, after two months, the annoying symptoms vanished.

And the next time I had a serious cold, after just three days of taking papain, I was symptom free.

Last summer, my Malaysian neighbor contracted dengue fever. Her Filipino housekeeper prepared a remedy made of papaya leaves. After washing the leaves and chopping them into small pieces, she crushed them in a mortar. Next, by hand, she squeezed out the leaf mass, and saved the poisonous looking, dark green liquid in a glass container. Three times a day, my neighbor took ten teaspoons of this extract. After three days, she was completely healthy again. And the list of benefits attributable to this vital bomb goes on.

Papaya and Science

Ever since Professor Luc Montagnier praised papaya's antioxidant properties publicly in 2001, the world of science has taken a keen interest in the exotic, tropical fruit. Even more so, because he prescribed it to Pope John Paul II, Ronald Reagan, and NASA astronauts. When asked about the fruit, he declared he gave the Pope fermented papaya in capsule form as a sign of his friendship. Later the media headlines read: "A Miracle! Pope's Complete Recovery!" However, the Vatican rushed to explain that the Pope never took the capsules. Whatever the case might have been in fact, over 250 research papers and 360 studies proving the antioxidant effects of papaya had already been published.

Papaya extract was officially acknowledged as a medicine by the FDA as early as 1982. The papaya tree, which is hardly ever subject to sickness or parasites, is armed with papain as its natural defense against destructive and disease causing microorganisms. It therefore seemed only logical to test its effect on humans. A large number of fundamental research papers and clinical trials have shown that the defense system is in fact transferable to humans. Papaya enzymes activate our defense cells as a protection against bacteria, fungus, viruses and even cancer cells. It is believed that science has yet to identify and define the entire scope of effective papaya substances. Despite the numerous studies mentioned above, papaya expert and University of Honolulu Professor Chung-Shih speaks of a virtual knowledge gap on the therapeutic value of the papaya plant.

Thanks to its wide range of benefits, papain has recently been added to the pharmacopoeias of a growing number of countries. While at least available in capsule form in Germany as an anti-ageing supplement, papain has not been approved as a medicine. "Further and more exact testing" is required. I am seriously wondering, whether this would be at all desirable for a certain industry?

Even in the mid-18th century, it was common knowledge that the milky papaya juice, known in German as "Latex", contained enzymes capable of breaking down proteins. However, it was not until the late 19th century, that its true value as a source of enzymes was recognized.

Here in South-East Asia, papain has long been the staple medicine prescribed by doctors for infectious diseases, for example.

Its immunity enhancing and balancing effect is simply breath-taking. Its antiviral, antibacterial and antifungal properties unburden our immune system, remove and even prevent the forming of immune complexes. To a layman, the medical term "immune complex" may sound positive, but this is highly deceptive. Immune complexes are formed by interlocking antigens and antibodies, which can attach to our tissue as a cluster and cause cell proliferation. Our body's phagocytes are not able to destroy these growths and as a result cause cancer and a number of other diseases.

Over the last few decades, our diet has changed fundamentally and, unfortunately, not to our advantage. We are ingesting far too many acidifying foods. Among them are all animal products such as processed and non-processed meat, fish, milk, eggs, yoghurt, cream cheese and cheese products. Also on the list are the many varieties of food containing sugar and refined wheat, not to mention all the processed and packaged foods with their countless chemical additives.

"Drink lots of milk, Sweetheart! It's good for your bones, because it's full of calcium", my mother often said to me. Certainly, most everyone is familiar with this phrase. The dreadful thing, unfortunately, is that it is false! The exact opposite is the case. A recent study shows that, in fact, milk, and all dairy products, actually deplete the calcium in our bodies, which contributes to mineral deficiencies, leading to hyperacidity. An acidic milieu is the ideal environment for bacteria, fungus and an array of diseases to develop, and in the worst case cancer, which thrives exclusively in an acidic environment.

Of all fruit known to us to date, the papaya is the most alkaline. This helps counteract acidification, thereby restoring our acid-alkaline balance. Simultaneously, it provides healthy intestinal flora and stimulates our metabolism. Our system's acid-alkaline levels are constantly under attack by modern, unhealthy and acidifying foods, along with medications and the stresses of modern living. As Paracelsus observed long ago, high acidity, or acidosis, is the primary cause of many diseases. Rheumatism, arteriosclerosis, diabetes and cancer are typical modern-day diseases caused by acidosis. Permanent hyperacidity often makes us suffer from depression and feel drained, fatigued, and irritable. A vicious cycle is set in motion when we use unhealthy substances, for instance coffee as a stimulant, alcohol to numb, and sugary foods to distract ourselves. These are the very foods and stimulants responsible for exacerbating acidity levels. We feel more and more stressed, our immune system gets weaker and weaker, which soon and often opens the gates to chronic and/ or serious illnesses.

Research on Papaya and Cancer

Cancer inhibiting substances have been discovered in the skin and leaves of papaya, as well as in the tree's stems. The American National Cancer Institute, NCI, has confirmed the papaya's effectiveness in battling cancer. Between 1992 and 1995, with NCI endorsement, Doctors Jerry L. McLaughlin, Yan Zhang, Qing Ye and Geng-Xian Zhao performed extensive studies at the Department of Medical Chemistry and Pharmacology on the effectiveness of papaya in treating cancer. Their in-depth studies led the researchers to unanimously conclude that "cancer-killing" substances were to be found in all parts of the papaya tree, especially in the leaves, stems and small branches.

In Australia, even the government gives out official information on papaya as a healing plant for cancer. Barbara Simonsohn, author of "Healing Power of Papaya", found a report dated as early as June 16th, 1906 in The British Medical Journal. In it, W. J. Branch describes how he succeeded in dissolving a tumor by injecting his patient with 2 grams of papain. "One of the tumors needed to be injected with the solution three times before disintegrating." What's impressive about this method, is that "the disintegration and dissolution process the enzymes initiate stops at the edges of the tumor." Normal, healthy cells are not affected or destroyed. The enzymes destroy the cancer, and only the cancer. Many famous scientists and doctors, among them Professor Chung-Shih Tang swear by the effectiveness of papain for cancer, attributing an especially important role to carpain, the main alkaloid found in papaya. American Dr. McLaughlin of the University of Lafayette in Indiana supports these findings and is equally convinced that carpain is a natural substance, capable of destroying cancer cells.

"We could reduce the cancer rate by fifty percent if we systematically treated potential cancer patients preventively with enzymes. Because prevention is everything. We must take into account that once the cancer has developed the majority of cancer patients do not succumb to their primary tumor, but rather to the ensuing metastatic spread. This is exactly what enzyme therapy is capable of preventing", says Viennese Professor Wrba.

Papaya enzymes have a multifactorial impact. For the Indians of Central and South America, the indigenous peoples of Australia and the Kahunas of Hawaii, the

"Guardians of Secrets", the fruit has been established for centuries as the traditional healing substance against cancer. There are numerous reports on people, long since considered hopeless by traditional medicine, whose lives were saved by the papaya. As of today, there are 600 scientific studies on the healing potential of papaya against this insidious illness.

The Aborigines make an anti-cancer drink out of papaya leaves. The first person ever to try this recipe was the Australian Stan Sheldon, who successfully fought his lung cancer with it. In 1962, he was diagnosed with a fast growing cancer in both lungs. Sheldon was deathly ill the day an old Aborigine gave him the secret papaya recipe a Shaman had taught him. Over a period of two months, Sheldon drank the brew, adding three teaspoons of molasses, which was another "healing secret". Two months later, the doctors found Stan Sheldon's lungs to be completely cancer free. He has been sharing his experience with other cancer patients ever since.

The proteolytic enzymes contained in papaya can reduce the side-effects of chemo and radiation therapy. In the sixties, the protective effect of papain against radiation was attested by the U.S. Airforce medical institute. During the course of radiation treatment, the papaya enzymes reduced and/or prevented diarrhea, skin rashes, mucous membrane swelling and tissue scaring. They ensured an accelerated elimination of inflammatory and metabolic waste products.

In a lecture given at the Habichtswald Clinic Oncology Department in 2001, Head Physician Dr. Wolfrum and Assistant Medical Director Dr. Mihai Palfi stated the following: "We have been able to prove the effectiveness of protective enzyme therapy for better tolerance of chemotherapy and radiation treatment. Radiation induced inflammation and edemas subside more quickly, radiation tolerance is improved, while the need for additional medication is decreased. Papaya enzymes now hold a firm place in the treatment of cancer, aging symptoms, digestive problems, and inflammation issues. Beside papain, the enzymes also contain useful beta-carotene, vitamin C, flavones and fibers such a pectin, essential oils, bitters and tannins. Papain enhances digestion and eliminates remaining protein residue from the intestinal walls, and is helpful against parasites, and good for a healthy intestinal flora."

According to Dr. Jerry McLaughlin, the active ingredients in papaya are a million times stronger than commonly used cytostatic drugs.

Since the ever growing number of reports from cancer survivors, healed thanks to treatment with fermented papaya leaf extract, the exotic fruit plays a significant role in cancer therapy and is increasingly generating interest in the medical field as well as the general public.

The Pharaohs' Medicine: Cinnamon

Would you have guessed that cinnamon can help lower your blood sugar levels? In the large box of pills Dr. K.S. gave me, there was a capsule called "Cinsulin with InSea2 and Crominex 3+". I went to see Doctor K. S. again, to ask him what Cinsulin was all about. And before answering my question, he gave me a very interesting lecture.

Presently, numerous tests and focused human studies have established the anti-diabetic properties of cinnamon, and clinical trials are causing considerable excitement among researchers world-wide. For over ten years, United States Department of Agriculture scientists studied this effect and found unambiguous data, clearly proving that blood sugar levels were lowered after just a two-month treatment with cinnamon. Also, cinnamon reduces the blood lipid and cholesterol levels, partly controlled by insulin - more specifically the "bad" LDL cholesterol - by up to 27 percent. Dr. K.S. told me that in India, shoe inlay soles were made and treated with 40 grams of finely ground cinnamon. This method allowed the spice to enter the body through the soles of the feet and regulate the human system. In Indian Ayurvedic Medicine, all parts of the cinnamon tree, from its leaves and bark to its roots, are used for healing purposes. Its leaves, for example, yield an oil which warms the body and is anti-inflammatory in colds and intestinal infections. Cinnamon therefore is not only used as a spice added to our beloved "Glühwein", (a European traditional winter and Christmas beverage, usually made of hot red wine, along with spices such as cinnamon, cloves, nutmeg, and sometimes raisins). It also stabilizes our circulation, lowers our blood pressure and dilates our blood vessels. Adding a pinch of cinnamon to coffee lessens its aggressive impact on the stomach.

Cinnamon is one of the oldest and most commonly used spices world-wide. In China it has been used as a medicine for over 4,000 years. Other advanced civilizations such as Ancient Rome and Greece, Mesopotamia, and Egypt, during the time of the Pharaohs, also included it in ceremonial rituals. Besides being regarded as a miracle remedy by the Ancient Greeks, it was an ingredient in the incense burned in their temples. The Egyptians valued its mummification properties as well as a remedy to ward off the flies attracted to their stored raw meat supplies.

Kansas State University researchers in Manhattan surely had heard of this method when they studied the antibacterial effect of cinnamon and published their findings in 2001. The spice has the ability to stop reproduction of bacteria commonly found in food. One trial on the effect of cinnamon, was done on standard, pasteurized commercial apple juice. The food microbiologists infected samples of the juice with salmonella, staphylococcus and Yersinia, three common kinds of bacteria. The comparison between the non-treated juice and the juice inoculated with cinnamon, showed a bacterial decrease in the cinnamon-apple juice within one to seven days. Likewise, the spice inhibited the development of coli bacteria and that not only in the juice but also in raw meat. No wonder the Ancient Egyptians burned cinnamon to protect their storage spaces.

Until the middle ages, extensive trade routes made the sweet smelling spice very costly and was often offered as a gift to popes and princes. In those days, it was prescribed mainly as a healing remedy for fever, colds, gynecological disorders, and digestive problems. While cinnamon grew increasingly popular as a spice in the late middle ages, its uses as a remedy receded into the background. In the 19th century, doctors were prescribing cinnamon for stomach and intestinal disorders. However, its anti-bacterial and anti-oxidant, its anti-fungal and anti-inflammatory properties as well as its spasmolytic qualities were not acknowledged before the mid 20th century. Cinnamon is further helpful against digestive problems, appetite loss, bloating and bowel gasses.

BY THE WAY: We like to use this wonderfully aromatic spice in our beverages, it is the perfect addition to refine our daily water rations. Simply add a cinnamon stick and some fresh mint leaves (optional) to a carafe of non-carbonated water.

We use it in many of our dishes as well, for instance, to give spinach a special zing. You should try it: add half or one teaspoon of cinnamon at most. Super delicious and very healthy.

Important Facts on Cinsulin

Avoiding carbohydrates is hardly possible in these fast-food times. This leads to an increase of glucose intolerance, and eventually, to diabetes. With age, our blood sugar levels tend to go up. Studies clearly show that cinnamon extract lowers the sugar levels in our blood. As prescribed by Dr. K. S., I take Cinsulin capsules three times a day – one before breakfast, one at 11:00 am and one 30 minutes before dinner. Of course this prescription is meant for me personally and should not be understood as the dosage for everyone!

Cinsulin is a food supplement, made of water and cinnamon. The cinnamon extract used in this case has been strongly cleansed and is highly water soluble. It can be taken to maintain healthy blood sugar levels as well as to enhance good health, general wellbeing and fitness. Cinsulin is not a medication! And yet, it has had an excellent effect on my health.

In a complex production process, a substance called coumarin is extracted from cinnamon. Up to ten years ago, the ingredient was said to cause liver damage and cancer. However, based on the safety evaluation by the European Food Safety Authority

(EFSA) on coumarin, which was updated in 2004, the following was stated: "The analysis of the most recent data on coumarin does not conclude that it has a cancer causing effect in humans." This is another great example of inconsistency – one day a substance is bad for us, the next day it's not. Coumarin is both a fragrance and a flavoring agent found in many plants, tonka beans and woodruff, for instance. While the more bitter tasting cassia variety of cinnamon is rich in coumarin, the milder Ceylon cinnamon barely contains the substance.

Teams of scientists worldwide have collected numerous data clearly proving the positive effect of Cinsulin on patients with adult-onset diabetes, also known as diabetes mellitus type 2. In 2011, the US Journal of Medical Food published the results of eight different clinical studies on Cinsulin done by the University of California and the Western Regional Research Center. The findings reconfirmed that Cinsulin is verifiably able to lower blood sugar levels in persons with type 2 diabetes or pre-diabetes. Throughout the study, all diabetic participants received their usual diabetes therapy. In addition, half the test subjects were given Cinsulin, while the other half were not. The diabetics treated with cinnamon capsules over a period of 90 days showed that their percentage of hemoglobin (HbA1c), a marker for high blood glucose, was significantly lower than that of the control group not given the cinnamon capsules. In my case, I was able to stop taking all diabetes medication after only ten months.

PLEASE NOTE: Because Cinsulin lowers your blood sugar levels, and in case you are on diabetes medication, you need to re-adjust the dose of the latter. You should definitely discuss this with your doctor. Should he not be open to alternative medicine, I suggest finding a reputable and competent practitioner in complementary medicine, rather than self-medicating and becoming your own guinea pig. The concept of complementary medicine entails a wide scope of methods applicable in addition to conventional medicine. The most famous among them are traditional Chinese medicine, homoeopathy, and phytotherapy, all of which have been practiced for thousands of years.

The Secret of Zen Monks: Matcha Tea

Especially here in Asia, people are generally well informed on healing herbs and alternative healing methods. Once, on a stormy afternoon, my Chinese neighbor served me a cup of matcha tea. "Here", she said, "something very special against stress and for a long life". Just the way she prepared it was enough to peak my interest in this tea - a poisonous looking green - which, by the way, was delicious. And ever since, I have it sent to me directly from a friend in Japan. It is there, or more precisely in Okinawa, that people live the longest and their longevity is attributed to their regular consumption of matcha tea.

A thousand years ago, one of the Zen monks' secrets to leading a long and stress-free life was drinking matcha tea! For 750 years, the secret tea remained the exclusive privilege of traditional tea ceremonies held by Japan's elite. Zen Master Eisai reveals the secret around matcha tea. "Tea has special life-prolonging powers. Wherever people cultivate tea, long life is ensured." The best quality tea is "koicha", meaning "thick", when translated. These tea leaves are over 30 years old. Also of good quality is "usucha" (thin). Its leaves are not quite as old and have a slightly bitter taste. My favorite tea is the "Uji matcha tea – koicha", originating from the Uji region in Japan. Ever since Master Eisai introduced matcha tea to Japan, Uji has been the prominent manufacturing center of this extraordinary tea. Not only is its taste especially delicate, it can perform virtual miracles.

Healing Tea from Ancient Times

Due to its many special properties, matcha tea is drawing growing attention worldwide. It stimulates our metabolism, can reduce stress, enhances our immune system, lowers cholesterol and has a rejuvenating effect. As opposed to black tea, matcha tea leaves are not fermented, allowing nearly all the beneficial substances of the plant to remain intact. These natural substances are not, as in other teas, replaced by flavoring agents.

Numerous tests have proven the effects of this far-eastern beverage. An eleven-year study (!), known as the Ohsaki Study, showed that it possesses actual life-prolonging qualities. According to the scientists involved, this is due to "its positive cardiovascular properties". This means our whole cardiovascular system is supported, including the heart, the coronary vessels as well as the entire arterial network. The study was conducted on 40,000 test subjects between the ages of 40 and 79. The mortality rate in the men's group dropped by 12 percent, whereas the women's rate dropped even further. It went down 23 percent.

One remarkable fact about matcha tea is its high antioxidant content. Catechins, as they are known in the jargon, are the substances contained in the tea which act as free radical interceptors in our bodies. "The green tea's ability to fight cancer turned out to be greater and more complex than science ever suspected", researchers declared at the University of Rochester Medical Center in the United States as early as 2003. They had discovered just how very rich the green tea was in antioxidants. There are 137 times more antioxidants in a single cup of matcha tea, than in a cup of common green tea. The tiny molecules are able to eliminate the carcinogenic toxins and chemicals found in tobacco. In short, this tea has unimaginable powers.

The Chinese and Japanese have been drinking match tea for many centuries. In Japan, it is an important part of the culture. In the 16th century, it was customary for feuding warlords to meet for a tea ceremony. Because the entrance of the tea house was very low, the enemy parties were forced to bow deeply to step inside. Everyone is equal in a tea house. Worldly leadership status is expected to be shed and left outside. This way, the adversaries were able to resume their dialog.

In the meantime, Hollywood had also discovered the slimming and rejuvenating tea. Stars like Meg Ryan, Amber Heard and top model Eva Padberg appreciate its qualities: "Because it makes you beautiful, keeps you young, and because it tastes so good."

Four weeks before the harvest, the tea plantations are covered with nets or bamboo matting. By reducing their exposure to sunlight, the leaves produce more chlorophyll. This not only causes them to turn that typically bright green and have a fine, fresh and slightly sweet taste, it also makes the leaves produce an array of substances beneficial to our health. The chlorophyll saturated leaves are hand-picked by farmers. They remove the leafstalks, midribs and veins. Next, they steam and dry the leaves, before finely pulverizing them in the traditional Japanese granite stone mill. In Uji, only the most valuable part of the leaf is used to manufacture matcha tea. It takes at least one hour to grind 3.5 ounces of leaves.

The preparation of this super tea is another feature that makes it stand out among all teas. Water heated to a temperature of 176° is poured into a bowl containing 3.5 to 7 ounces (1/2 -3/4 tsp.) of the fine powder. Now a light touch is needed. With a so-called "chasen", a very fine whisk, carved out of a single piece of bamboo, the brew is whisked on the surface to form bubbles. The foamier the tea, the better. The trick is to whisk with the chasen in a back and forth movement, in an "M" pattern. It works best, when the little bamboo whisk is moistened beforehand. I place it in the bowl containing the powder and add the hot water. Once I have spread the tea lightly on the bottom of the bowl, I start whisking and the chasen may no longer touch the bottom.

How Matcha Tea Aids Weight Loss

Matcha tea contains approximately 2 to 4 percent caffeine. Other green teas contain under 3 percent on average. With regular teas, the beverage is made only of an extract, while Matcha tea consists of the entire pulverized leaf.

A U.S. study found that matcha tea drinkers absorb three times the amount of the secondary plant substance called EGCG (Epigallocatechin gallate) than people consuming other kinds of tea. Numerous health benefits are attributed to EGCG. It is believed to be anti-inflammatory, to have a positive impact on immune system diseases and health promoting influences on cancer afflictions. "It seems to inhibit tumor growth", scientists say. Even in Alzheimer research, studies on

EGCG are being conducted. Researchers assume that this high quality tea is able to stop the disease in its early stages.

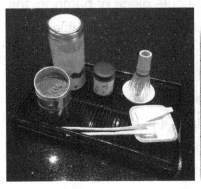 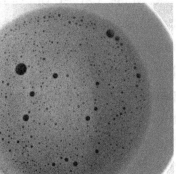

The EGCG ingredient is ideal for dieting. Several cups of matcha tea, on a daily basis, over a longer period of time, will cause weight loss - specifically through fat breakdown. It is also said to reduce fat storage.

Matcha tea is also believed to be able to lower the so-called bad LDL cholesterol. The study verifying this fact was published in the U.S. Journal of Clinical Nutrition in 2011. It was proven that the intake of Matcha tea clearly regulated the body's cholesterol balance. Furthermore, the tea enhances thermogenesis, which is the generation of body heat through metabolism and helps the body's fat burning process to get into really high gear.

Thermogenesis burns off excess energy and is transformed into body heat. A well-functioning metabolism is a very important companion on the road to a dream figure.

Matcha tea is known to be especially effective after sports by helping to burn off 25 percent more calories.

The potent green tea contains up to five times more L-Theanine than found in common green teas. L-Theanine is an amino acid found in both green as well as black tea leaves. As opposed to caffeine, L-Theanine has a calming effect, by activating the brain's alpha waves, thereby reducing stress, enhancing relaxation, and lowering blood pressure.

Even though matcha tea contains caffeine, the relaxing effect of L-Theanine balances out the caffeine. This is how a cup of the Japanese tea enhances concentration and clarity of mind without the nervousness caused by an excessive consumption of coffee. In the afternoon, a cup of matcha tea can do wonders when you feel the need for an energy boost or a pick-me-up.

For some time now, even Baumkuchen with matcha tea filling - deliriously delicious - and many other newer foods and drinks made with matcha tea have been available on the market. (*Baumkuchen* is a traditional German Christmas pastry, in the form of a round layer cake with a hole in the middle, from being baked on a spit. The typical rings that appear when sliced resemble tree growth rings, hence the German name, *Baumkuchen*, which means "tree cake". The cake is often refined with various fillings such as marzipan, almonds, pistachios or rum.)

INCIDENTALLY: Please buy this tea in organic health food stores to be sure it has been grown without artificial fertilizers, herbicides, or chemical plant protection products. Never pour boiling hot water directly on the matcha powder, it can make it taste "grassy". First, boil the water and let it sit for about five minutes before using it to brew the tea. Personally, I like to sweeten my tea with half a teaspoon coconut flower sugar. And these days, the absolute number one on our dessert hit-parade list is matcha tea ice-cream (see pages 225 and 257).

Three Tiny Seeds with Super (Man) Powers

"Like coconut oil, chia, amaranth and quinoa seeds also have the ability to burn belly fat", Doctor K.S. declared in one of our many sessions. Burn belly fat? He did not have to tell us twice. We immediately bought all these little kernels and started experimenting with them.

As small as they are, any other seed variety would turn green with envy if they knew what powers are hidden in chia seeds. Even the world of science was speechless, once this treasure made its reappearance and unveiled all its highly valuable ingredients. Hollywood now considers these superfoods the secret recipe for beauty, good health, and slimming. Chia seeds leave you feeling satisfied for long a long time and thereby supports excess weight loss. Thanks to their high content in soluble fiber, the metabolizing process of carbohydrates is drawn out over a longer period of time, which essentially curbs your appetite.

Meanwhile, stars like Sharon Stone, Oprah Winfrey and Miranda Kerr swear by this new mega-nutrition (which is actually ancient) and is currently gaining in popularity all over Europe.

Recently Rediscovered: Chia Seeds

The story of these tiny seeds goes all the way back to the Aztecs, Mayans, and the South-Western Native Americans. The small black or white seeds, full of proteins, were the staple food and healing ingredients of all of these ancient cultures. "Chia", in Mayathan, the classic Mayan language, means "strength". The seeds were mainly used to provide high-energy. Carried in small pouches during a messenger mission, the seeds gave the Native American couriers incredible energy boosts along the way. Aztec warriors needed only a daily ration of two tablespoons of soaked chia seeds to survive and infuse them with mystical and super natural powers. It is a proven fact, that chia seeds were a staple food as early as 3,500 years before Christ. Between 1,500 and 900 B.C., the seeds served as currency and were leveed as a yearly tax from conquered nations. The Aztecs are known to have pleased their Gods with them, using them as the base for their face and body painting during ritual ceremonies. By developing unique cultivation techniques, the Aztecs were very advanced in agriculture. Using the knowledge their ancestors, the Tolteks, had passed along, they turned lakes and other wetlands into solid, arable land in the vicinity of their housing. They wove large mats out of tree bark and reeds and fastened them to the banks of shallow waters. The matting was then covered with lake sediment and used as acreage to plant not only chia, but also amaranth, beans, and corn. These islands were known as "hanging gardens" or "chinampas". Originally, these hanging gardens were created out of the necessity to provide sufficient nourishment for the densely populated Aztec community.

Hollywood celebrities cherish the tiny seeds for their high content in omega-3 fats, vitamin E and their antioxidant properties, which ensure firm and elastic skin, prevent wrinkles, and enhance mental concentration. The chia seed's swelling ability is impressive, it makes them very filling even though they are low in calories. When soaked in water, they swell into a clear, gelatinous mass within ten minutes. The great thing is, this enables them to store large amounts of water, thereby keeping our bodies sufficiently hydrated, especially during physical exertion. This super food not only contributes to our good looks, it also flushes disease-causing bacteria out of our intestines. Like a virtual digestion-broom, the gelatinous mass sweeps through the gastro-intestinal tract, supporting the elimination of intestinal deposits and regulates bowel movement. Holistic nutrition experts are growing increasingly enthusiastic about the little food bombs as sustainable sources of high energy and as digestive enhancers. The Aztecs and Mayans knew of their ability to bind and eliminate dangerous toxins and acids from the body long ago. Furthermore, chia seeds are gluten-free and perfect for persons suffering from gluten intolerance. By building a barrier between ingested carbohydrates and digestive enzymes, they have a positive impact on blood sugar levels. The process of transforming carbohydrates into sugar is slowed down, causing nutritional energy to reach the body at a slower pace and, as a result, to be more sustainable for a longer period of time. This effect is beneficial to diabetics and athletes alike, as well as for anyone having to mind their cholesterol levels. It is their high content in soluble fiber, which allows chia seeds to help regulate cholesterol balance. The little miracle kernels are also believed to possess hormone regulating, immune system boosting, and muscle repairing properties. No other grain can compete with the nutritional density of these mini-seeds, abundantly rich in vitamin B, iron, calcium, potassium, copper, niacin, phosphorus, thiamine, riboflavin and zinc. The plant contains 38 percent oil and 23 percent protein - which is far more than is found in rice, corn, wheat or barley. All this supports healthy tissue development, especially important during pregnancy.

Chia plants are extremely unpopular among insects, making the use of pesticides unnecessary. Their highly oily leaves serve as a natural shield to ward off insects.

The omega-3 and omega-6 fatty acid imbalance, which many Germans suffer from, can also be regulated by chia seeds, by delivering the perfect balance of the two omega fatty acids. Using the seeds as an omega-3 source can contribute to the preservation of worldwide fish populations. In Central Mexico, in some Latin American countries, and in Australia, chia seeds are grown as chicken feed, to enrich the eggs with omega-3 fatty acids.

In September, the weed-like, annual plant spreads tufts of magical blue carpeting across the fields of Central Mexico. In the fall, the almost insipid yet nutritious and versatile seeds are harvested. Whether added to jams or marmalades, drinks and desserts, to salads, soups, sauces, biscuits, muffins and cakes or sprinkled on fried eggs or a slice of bread, they enrich a healthy diet and can be used to replace certain foods, such as eggs and flour! The possibilities are virtually endless. Since most chia bread recipes require only a relatively small amount, I developed my own recipe. It tastes wonderful and has great firm consistency (see recipe "Katharina's Chia Bread" page 266).

The Astonishing Nutritional Content of the Chia Seed

Chia seeds contain nearly six times the amount of calcium in comparison to that of whole milk, twice as much potassium as in bananas, and they outrank blue berries and goji berries with three times the amount of antioxidants. 3.5 oz. of chia seeds deliver as many antioxidants as 31.7 oz. of oranges! The "runner's food" score is especially high regarding its protein content. Compared to beans, chia seeds have five times the amount, and twice as much protein as any other kind of grain or seed. They are also eight times richer in omega-3 than salmon.

They leave spinach far behind with six times the amount of iron in them and five times the amount of folic acid.

The first person to discover the excellent properties of these seeds was a University of Arizona research Professor, who was searching for alternatives for Argentina's agriculture. His first analysis produced such astonishing results that he immediately decided to dedicate his work to researching the little seeds, so that all of humanity might profit from their immense health benefits. For over 25 years, Dr. Wayne Coats has been researching this unique plant and has even developed special techniques and machinery to optimize harvest results. Due to his passionate enthusiasm for the super food, he has been nick-named Mr. Chia. Another passion of his is marathon running, during which he always carries his runner's food in a film roll container to re-fill on energy and increase his endurance. In 2005, "Mr. Chia", aka Wayne Coates, and Richard Ayerzaco wrote a book called "Chia: Rediscovering a Forgotten Crop of the Aztecs". Later, in 2012, he published another book titled "Chia: The Complete Guide to the Ultimate Superfood".

Chia Seeds: Quality is Vital!

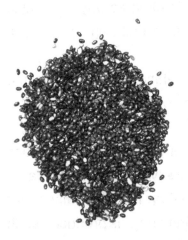

You can tell good quality seeds by their color. They should be either consistently black or white. If they are brown, this means they are not fully ripe and are less rich in oil, protein, omega-3 fats etc. Sometimes even traces of weeds and plant parts are found in the mix. You can perform your own quality test, by soaking one teaspoon of seeds in 12 teaspoons of filtered water in a glass. You can use a little more water, but not too much. Let it sit for approximately 20 minutes. If the chia seeds completely absorb all of the water, you can be certain to have ripe and best quality seeds. If, however, there are still some floating on the water surface, this indicates that there are too many unripe seeds, which do not properly absorb the water and is a sign of lesser quality. Before buying, be sure to choose good quality seeds.

The Incan Miracle Grain: Amaranth

On the list of foods Dr. K.S. gave me for my blood type, I saw the word "amaranth". I had never even heard the word in my life, nor was I aware that it is the name for one of the healthiest Inca grains and one of the oldest crops in the world. I was enthralled and read everything I could find on amaranth and especially recipes that would show me all the delicious dishes I could create with it. Whether sweet or savory, thanks to its versatility, the cooking possibilities of amaranth are endless. We eat it instead of rice, potatoes or pasta. I even dared baking bread with amaranth. My family was delighted with my very first amaranth meatballs, which I even served my father while on a family visit back home in Germany. I'd like to add here, that my father normally wouldn't touch "any of this newfangled stuff" and believes "it's all nonsense". His meal credo is: On Sundays, a decent piece of meat belongs on the table! Consequently, I convinced my mother to keep secret that "my" meatballs (called "Bouletten" in the Rhineland region where my parents live) were not made of meat at all. He ate them with great pleasure. Once our secret was revealed, he was very surprised. What? No meat? Nope, just amaranth!

Amaranth was also cultivated by the Aztecs in the Central and South American highlands and was equally considered a precious "gold". Even though the tiny kernel is rich in healthy components such as iron, protein, fats and large amounts of minerals like calcium, zinc, and magnesium, we Europeans were initially hardly interested in the "holy Incan miracle grain". And this despite the fact that the seeds are a wonderful culinary addition and have multiple gifts to offer. In Germany, this has been an insider tip for some time now. Thanks to its multiple uses in modern wholefood cooking, there are many good reasons for adding amaranth to our menus on a regular basis. Popped amaranth is crunchy, with a slightly nutty taste. In combination with honey and nuts, it is part of the traditional South American sweet called "Alegria".

Amaranth is not only rich in nutrients, it is easily digested, making it perfect for mothers to feed their babies during the transition of weaning. Astronauts are known to use this "power pack" on their long journeys into space. Also athletes use it shortly before a competition, thanks to its lightness. The grains deliver instant, sustainable energy, as opposed to the isolated sugars contained in most industrial athletes' products, which vanish fairly quickly.

Until the 16th century, the amaranth plant was virtually unknown. Spanish conquerors discovered it while exploring the new American continent. Besides corn and beans, amaranth was a staple food for the Incas and Aztecs living there, and they used it in religious ceremonies such as ritual human sacrifice. While massacring thousands during their conquests, the Spanish also outlawed cultivation and consumption of amaranth under penalty of death. And yet, the miracle plant survived.

Amaranth was to know a revival in South America 400 years later, and, along with 70 varieties of the species, spread to almost all corners of the globe. Amaranth is cultivated not only in Mexico and the Andes, but also by mountain tribes in India, Pakistan and Nepal, as well as in West Africa. It is even farmed in California and in the southern states of the US. In Indonesia, the plant leaves are much appreciated as a kind of spinach green.

Compared to other grain species, amaranth contains much higher levels of protein and fat. Even though it has cereal-like properties and can be used in similar ways, the healthy plant does not strictly belong to the cereal species, but rather to the foxtail plant variety, which are pseudo-cereals, or pseudo-grains.

After pollination, tiny, lentil-shaped seeds appear on the underside of the amaranth leaf, hardly a millimeter in diameter. One thousand of these tiny seeds, which are smaller than mustard kernels, barely weigh 0.035 oz. After a ripening period of 4 to 5 months, they are harvested and laid out in the sun to dry.

One single plant delivers approximately 50,000 very small and very light-weight seeds. For 0.035 oz,

1,500 seeds must be gathered by hand. And despite their small size, they have much to offer. Because the seedling in the grain is proportionally much larger than its endosperm, it is able to store all the valuable components inside it. With approximately 18 percent protein (!), the "miracle grain" is very much at the top of the winners' list and is the protein-richest "cereal" of them all. Its high protein content makes amaranth especially valuable for vegetarians, who primarily draw their protein supply from plants. The same goes for its relatively high iron content.

One of the fatty acids found in amaranth is the double bond unsaturated linoleic acid, which regulates our cholesterol levels.

Its high fiber content stimulates bowel movement, thereby ensuring healthy digestion and counteracting constipation. Because its fiber keeps you satisfied for longer periods of time, it helps with weight loss.

Thanks to its high nutritional density, the grain is particularly suitable for the elderly, whose appetite tends to decrease with age, even though their nutritional needs remain the same. Regular amaranth consumption is said to help with chronic headaches and migraines, strengthen our respiratory tracts, slow down the aging process and alleviate sleeping problems.

For people who must avoid wheat, rye, barley and oats, due to gluten intolerance, this Inca wheat is especially valuable since, as opposed to all grains mentioned above, amaranth is gluten free.

The lack of gluten's sticky properties in amaranth may cause problems when baking, which can easily be remedied by adding thickening agents such as locust bean gum to the dough.

Little Power Kernels: Quinoa

On our list, I found another word completely unknown to me: quinoa. Just between the two of us, until now I had always considered myself to be fairly well educated. But in the course of my many sessions with Dr. K.S. and the research these sessions prompted me to look into, I started to suspect otherwise. With the exception of various articles in the media, which, looking back, turned out to be either half-heartedly researched, often senselessly dissected and sometimes blatantly false, I felt I knew absolutely nothing about healthy nutrition. Not to say that I think of myself as the font of all knowledge, I can draw on personal experience and now say that I know far more about healthy eating and health enhancing foods than ever before. And undisputed scientific research confirms all I have come to know.

For thousands of years, quinoa and amaranth alike have been cultivated in the Andes highlands, at over 13,000 ft., which is too high an elevation for corn to grow. The so-called Peruvian rice was a staple food for the Incas, and also served as a remedy for sore throats.

Quinoa contains all nine essential amino acids and is considered one of the best vegetable protein sources.

In 2013, UN Secretary General Ban Ki Moon declared: "Thanks to its specific advantages, and especially in these times of climate change, this plant can help fight hunger in the world."

Quinoa is gluten-free and, like amaranth, surpasses our commonly known cereal varieties by far. It is not a true cereal, but rather a member of the botanical goosefoot family and is therefore more closely related to spinach, beet roots and chard.

The one-year-old quinoa plant reaches a height of over six feet. The seed color varies from red to white to black. Harvesting them is a little difficult, because they do not all ripen simultaneously. As is the case with Amaranth, this requires manual harvesting. Compared to wheat, quinoa contains two and a half times more fat, consisting mainly of unsaturated, long-chain fatty acids. This vegetable alpha-linolenic acid is a poly-unsaturated omega-3 fatty acid, normally found only in fish. What's more, quinoa is abundant in calcium, magnesium, iron and zinc, as well as being a great source of vitamin E and vitamins of the B group. Also quinoa is wholesome for people with a lactose sensitivity. Basically, it offers our systems much the same health benefits as amaranth does - with the exception of infants under the age of two and for anyone with intestinal inflammation or gastroenteritis. Why? Because quinoa protects itself against pests with saponins, a bitter tasting compound, which can cause damage to the walls of not yet fully developed or inflamed intestines.

This is also the reason why the seeds should be thoroughly rinsed under hot running water before cooking. For older children and grown-ups, eating quinoa is normally not a problem at all.

Red Hot Chili Peppers

Time and again people ask me: "Do you actually eat foods as spicy hot as the South-East Asians do?"

"Yes, I do. And I love it", is my answer.

At first, it burns like hell in your mouth, then you get "hot flashes". Such are the typical symptoms during a meal spiced with chili. Here in South-East Asia, in many dishes, chili peppers are widely used - sometimes more, sometimes less. Many food stands and restaurants serve little green peppers as a welcoming amuse-gueule before almost every dish. Incidentally, red chili peppers are spicier than the green ones and the smaller they are, the hotter. But actually, the spicy peppers are just pretending. In reality, they do not damage your taste buds nor any inner organs. On the contrary, this solanaceous, or nightshade plant, is one of the healthiest foods of all. This means chili peppers are healthy spice bombs. Ever since chili peppers found their way into Christopher Columbus' luggage and were brought back from South America around 500 years ago, this plant, which is related to the rather unspectacular bell pepper, is considered a culinary enrichment. In the 17th century, Portuguese missionaries introduced the chili pepper to Thai cuisine. Capsaicin is the ingredient which makes it hot and spicy. By causing the nervous system to perceive burning, the body reacts by producing endorphins, the pain soothing hormones which are also well known for making us feel happy. Fresh chili peppers contain two to three times as much vitamin C as in the same amount of citrus fruit, but of course it would be impossible to consume the same amount of chili peppers. Not only do they contain vitamins B1, B2, B6, B12 and beta carotene, but also many valuable minerals such as potassium, calcium, magnesium, phosphorus, and zinc. So it is not surprising that chili peppers have established a lasting reputation for having any number of health enhancing effects.

In case you're thinking about increasing your intake of chili peppers now, you don't have to worry about the burning effect. Even though a glass of milk my help, due to the milk protein which counteracts the spiciness, I recommend removing all the little white seeds in the pepper before eating them. This is the best way to reduce the burning.

Salt of the Earth

"Could it be, that all the new salt varieties recently offered on the market affect our health in different ways?", I asked Dr. K.S. one day. I had been thinking about this for some time now, and I really wanted to know the truth about our favorite kind - sea salt. "Oh, definitely", was his short answer, again followed by an interesting lecture.

Although, as opposed to common, refined table salt, sea salt is still the preferable alternative. However, it can, unfortunately, also have traces of heavy metals and lead, due to seawater pollution. Yet, it is still much healthier than normal, refined table salt, which is processed with chemicals such as aluminum compounds to make it easy to sprinkle.

The even healthier alternatives are rock (pink Himalaya) and crystal salts, which "ripen" under the pressure of a mountain for centuries and, known as "white gold", were once accessible only to nobility.

Most of the trace elements and minerals found in crystal salt are finely dispersed in so-called colloidal form. The difference between rock salt and crystal salt is much like the difference between a crystallized quartz and a brook stone. But as pure, natural products, both salts are virtually pollutant free.

Thanks to a built-in regulatory system, we are not likely to over-dose on natural salts like Himalaya salt. According to Dr. K.S., tinctures of salt brine are very effective in restoring PH balance by regulating electrolyte levels naturally. Crystal salt baths also support detoxification of our bodies, our immune system and are known to work miracles on neurodermatitis, acne, and joint diseases such as rheumatism.

Iodine rich table salt has basically become a no-go for causing any number of allergies and because of its damaging side effects. Table salt, which undergoes a refining process with various chemicals and bleaching components, should no longer appear on any shopping list, especially if it is meant for cooking. A human's basic need for salt is 0.21 - 0.42 ounces, the amount healthy kidneys are able to process. Excessive salt intake causes a fiendish theft: in order to isolate and dissolve the excess salt, the system needs abundant amounts of water, which it must "steal" from somewhere. It takes it out of our cells! Without this life-sustaining water, in other words, without their cell water, the cells die off. Imagine a beautiful flower or any plant that died due to lack of water. It's the same with our cells, when they absorb large quantities of the wrong salt.

Bamboo Salt: Buddhist Spice and Healing Remedy

A lot of knowledge in Europe - if we think of Hildegard von Bingen - and in Asia alike, goes back to the ancient wisdom of monks. In Buddhist monasteries, food was not so much a matter of material substances but was rather seen as a means to gain spiritual fulfillment, harmony and good health with the help of the ethereal energies in the food. For diversity, the monks used only the best of salts, for they not only knew of its ability to refine their dishes, but, more importantly, of its health benefits. Over a thousand years ago, they filled bamboo canes with sun-dried sea salt, sealing one end with yellow clay. The salt was then burned at high temperatures for 24 hours, leaving behind a sort of salt "pad", which in turn was ground up and replaced inside the bamboo pipe. Again, the burning process was repeated eight times in a row. The ninth time, the monks would add pine resin to the fire as an accelerant, raising the temperature to 2,192 degrees. It was not until this procedure of repeatedly melting and cooling that the salt reached its perfect quality. They called it bamboo salt.

Still today, this "perfect" salt is used for detoxification in cases of inflamed gastro-intestinal ulcers, digestive problems, liver disease, kidney stones and diabetes. Salt that has been burned nine times has distinctly higher antioxidant powers than the one with only two or three burning procedures. Its PH value is approximately ten to eleven, giving it a strong alkaline quality, thanks to its many alkaline minerals, among them especially iron, potassium, magnesium, silicon and zinc. Also the yellow clay plays an important role. It offers numerous health benefits as a healing earth by binding and cleansing the body of toxic substances. The special properties of bamboo salt can protect us from the many environmental and nutritional pollutants we are unwittingly exposed to on a daily basis. To detox, says Dr. K.S., on an empty stomach, drink 0.52 pints of non-carbonated water, at room temperature, mixed with a teaspoon of Himalaya salt. Or, "If you have trouble drinking salt water, you can take the teaspoon of salt directly into your mouth and quickly rinse it down with the prescribed amount of water." Be sure, however, to be near a toilette in the next few hours! Note that this procedure is not permitted for dialysis patients or anyone with acute kidney disease!

The Divine Monk Fruit: Luo Han Guo

According to legend, in south east China, as early as the 13th century, Luohan monks cultivated an extraordinary plant which crowns its yearly growth with a very special fruit known as luo han guo. For many long centuries, along with the know-how of its complicated cultivation, the Zhuang-Zu minority living there at the time, kept the health benefits of this fruit, belonging to the gourd family, a secret. This explains the monk fruit's late entry into Traditional Chinese Medicine. However, as knowledge of the fruit's uses began to spread and sales increased explosively throughout the Zhuang-Zu community, its cultivation capacity reached its limit by 1900. Rare and highly nutritious, the fruit, sometimes also spelled luo-han-guo, flourishes only on mountain sides and under very specific climate conditions. Considered a rare specialty to this day, the Chinese believe in its power to promote longevity.

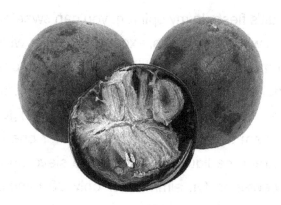

The divine monk fruit is popular for its sweet taste and its medicinal healing properties for coughs, sore throats and lung problems. It is a natural sweetener, 300 times sweeter than beet or cane sugar and the ideal replacement for commonly used sugar.

BY THE WAY: I tried monk fruit myself, and I love it. Recently, I have been using it as a sweetener and even produced my own version of a diet cola, which is much healthier and keeps my blood sugar levels in balance.

When cooked, the round, slightly fuzzy, green brown fruit yields a dark red, brownish liquid. Chinese herbal markets offer either the whole fresh fruit or the dried version. Since the mid-nineties, luo han guo extract has become a commercial product. As mentioned before, the juice is used for respiratory problems and diabetes. I became curious as to whether or not it may be a better alternative to other sweeteners such as stevia, of which I am not a fan. My answer is yes. The sweetness is due to the glycosides - a certain type of mogrosides - contained in the fruit's flesh. In my opinion, you can sweeten most any drink with luo han guo, except for coffee, which I do not recommend. But for baking and preparing desserts, the Buddha fruit, as it is also known, is ideal. It is easily prepared: wash and break apart three luo han guo balls and let them simmer in a pint of water for one hour at most. Strain the liquid through a fine sieve and use it as a sweetener. Or, simmer for only 30 minutes and serve as tea. To convert sugar quantities to luo han guo powder, simply divide the sugar figure by 200. If, for instance, a recipe requires 100 grams of sugar, you will need only 0.5 grams of powder, depending on the powder's concentration, which you can taste to determine. The pressed powder in tab form is more easily measured. The sweetener is also available on the Internet in liquid form.

A Scientific Look at the "Sweet Round Fruit"

It wasn't until the 20th century that luo han guo gradually became well-known outside of China. In 1938, Professor George Weidman Groff and Hoh Hin Cheung mentioned its effects in an unpublished manuscript, written in English. "[It is] Often used as the main ingredient in cooling drinks, that is to say drinks for the purpose of lowering fevers or counteracting other physical ailments, or as a cooling beverage in hot weather." Groff writes further, that while visiting the US Department of Agriculture in 1917, botanist Frederick Coville showed him the luo han guo seeds he had purchased in a local Chinese store in Washington D.C. Later, in 1941, he found the originals, along with a botanical description, in a store in San Francisco. And that's when research on the "sweet round fruit" began. The National Geographic Society gave G.W. Groff and Walter Tennyson Swingle of the Department of Agriculture a grant to research the plant.

Here in the Tropics, the round fruit is often added to summer drinks. The luo han guo fruit drink, served either hot or cold, is ideal for quenching thirst and preventing overheating. Because it is low in calories and has a low glycemic index (GI), it is also suitable for diabetics. The Chinese use it mostly to sooth weak or dry lungs, to break up persistent phlegm, to cure coughs, breathing problems, and whooping cough, and to treat sore throats, tonsillitis or pharyngitis, as well as constipation and sunstroke. The round fruit is also used to make tea or is added to stews and rice porridges.

The perennial monk fruit is rich in protein, vitamin C and 26 inorganic elements such as iron, nickel, selenium, tin, iodine and others. The fruit, either fresh or dried, undergoes a pulverization process, extracting 80 percent natural sweetener.

Several studies on mice and rats show that the mysterious fruit can possibly play an important role in the treatment of diabetes and its related cardiovascular damages as well as protecting the pancreas. Researchers further concluded that the extract of this fruit can have a calming effect on asthma and allergies. A Japanese study on mice in 2003, showed that the fruit's mogrosides had a "noteworthy inhibitory effect" on skin cancer. This lead the researchers to consider the possibility of a correlation between sugar consumption and the risk of cancer.

The common disadvantage of all these studies is that they are not human studies, and this leaves a big question mark regarding luo han guo. However, the experiments we have today are promising. And one thing is certain, in China, the "divine monk fruit" has been used as a medicine for hundreds of years. The fine hairs on the fruit shell are used to heal wounds, whereas boils and psoriasis are removed with the help of its ground-up roots. Its extract is good for edema and cerebral edema treatment, extensive burn injuries, acute kidney failure and glaucoma. Furthermore, the fruit is believed to support the immune and glandular system, the digestive and the respiratory tracts.

The oldest production site is the Yongfou Pharmaceutical Factory in Guangxi, China. Here the dried fruit is sold as an ingredient in herbal brews to be used for treating various respiratory diseases.

For usage in the western part of the world, real monk fruit sweetener can be found on the internet. Be sure to read the tab or liquid labeling closely, because as soon as there is a run on a natural product, certain producers become very creative.

The American FDA classified the round fruit as safe, declaring it a GRAS-product (Generally Recognized as Safe). Procter and Gamble patented a process for sweetener production as early as 1995. As described in the patent application, although the fruit itself is sweet, it contains too many other aromas, making it unsuitable for use as a sweetener on a larger scale. P & G therefore developed a process to eliminate the undesirable aromas. For longer preservation, and to remove the unwanted flavors from the fresh fruit, it is slowly dried in ovens. This process however, also creates a bitter taste, which is obviously one reason for the modest success of the P & G product on the market. In the P & G process, the fresh fruit is picked BEFORE it is ripe, letting it ripen during storage. Next, the skin and seeds are removed and the remains crushed to make a concentrated juice or puree suitable for food production.

I cooked the RIPE fruit, INCLUDING the seeds and carefully washed skin. The taste was delicious and I am able to use the concentrate in many ways.

Not Only for Whales: The Potency of Krill

Krill, in Norwegian, means "whale food" because whales are mostly found wherever there are large swarms of krill. It is also the main source of nutrition for penguins, seals, icefish, squid, the albatross and other birds. Because Antarctic krill is very rich in Omega-3 fats, it has become increasingly important not only to the food industry but also to alternative medicine, the cosmetic and pharma industries, as well as to fish farming as feed.

In the seventies, one of Germany's ministers of research even proposed using krill to solve the world hunger problem. Once informed, India's government took steps to tackle its malnutrition issues with the help of the tiny crustaceans. But processing krill turns out to be highly problematic. It must be cleaned and shock frozen as quickly as possible to prevent it from spoiling.

On the other hand, krill has the advantage of being at the bottom of the food chain, living exclusively on phytoplankton and not being polluted with pesticides and heavy metals, as is the case with so many other marine species. Krill cannot be farmed and can only be brought up from the depths of very clean waters.

This shrimp-like, luminescent crustacean is especially valuable to us due to its richness in omega-3 fats, which our body is unable to produce on its own. Fatty fish, such as salmon, mackerel and tuna are the only other sources with comparable omega-3 fatty acids. These are very important for our health since they can help with inflammation, ensure normal blood pressure, healthy cholesterol, and blood clotting balance. So it is no wonder that krill oil ranks highly on the list of superfoods. Chemical analyses show that, as phospholipid-bound fatty acids, the omega-3 fatty acids of krill oil are especially easy for us to assimilate. Fish oil, on the other hand, is much harder for us to metabolize due to the fact that it is bound to triglycerides. Thanks to its richness in antioxidants, high quality krill oil is also sustainable for longer periods of time.

"Could this oil be the solution to restoring an omega-fatty acid imbalance and to fighting the inflammations caused by this imbalance?", I asked Dr. K.S. during one of our sessions. And which krill oil should I choose? The market is flooded with all kinds of krill oil with any number of ingredients and advertising promises.

Studies show differences in both quality and in the actual effects of varying krill oils. Krill oil does not always actually contain what is promised on the label.

So, how do I find the best possible krill oil?

According to Dr. K.S., the one to pick should have the highest omega-3 concentration, and the fatty acids should be bound in phospholipid form as opposed to triglyceride form. High quality products make this distinction on their labels and brochures.

The phospholipid form makes it easier for our systems to absorb larger quantities of omega-3 fatty acids instead of eliminating them without absorbing them. When bound to triglycerides, the actual intake of omega-3 fatty acids remains very low. Imagine going to the gas station for 13 gallons of gasoline for your car, but only 10 percent go into your tank, and 90 percent spill into the gutter. However, at the check-out, you are still required to pay for the entire 13 gallons. That seems unfair, doesn't it? This is comparable to what happens in our bodies when we use the "wrong" oil. Phospholipids, on the other hand, ensure that all the beneficial fatty acids reach the vitally important organs, such as our brain, heart and joints. The components of krill oil not only support our heart and arteries; studies show that they help lower the risk of dangerous disease such as vascular constriction, which often lead to heart attack. They also reduce the risk of brain inflammation, which can be caused by an omega-6 and omega-3 imbalance. All this to say that krill oil ensures good brain function, even in old age. Krill oil is very expensive. I recommend buying only the best quality oil.

Thanks to their positive influence on hormone balance as well as on inflammation, the omega-3 fatty acids in krill oil have been proven to be beneficial during PMS (pre-menstrual syndrome). In one study conducted, a group of 70 women was divided into two groups, each of which were given either one gram of fish oil, or one gram of krill oil for three months. At pre-determined dates, the women were asked to fill out a standardized questionnaire, gathering data on their physical and emotional ailments. Both groups showed significant improvement in their symptoms. However, the krill-group needed far less pain medication.

Another study compared the effects of krill oil as opposed to those of fish oil on blood fat levels. Fish oil as well as krill oil both improved the blood fat levels examined. Cholesterol balance was improved; the "bad" LDL cholesterol and triglycerides levels went down, and the "good" HDL cholesterol levels were elevated. Although the krill oil in the one-gram dosage was demonstrably superior to the fish oil, experts found the results to be controversial. The European Food and Safety Authority (EFSA) conclusion was even harsher: "Upon examination of promotional statements implying health benefits, we conclude that no cause and effect has been proven." On the other hand, this same authority sees no reason to ban dangerous trans fats from our food.

Plant Pigment Against Belly Fat: Chlorophyll

One day, friends of ours told us of a plan in Germany to introduce a "veggie-day", and the controversy this was causing. It seemed rather ridiculous for us here in Malaysia, almost as if compulsory vegan diets were being instated. We also had our doubts about individuals actually sticking to this rule, because humans will not let the law dictate their diets, and rightly so. On the other hand, if the government were to join in by reducing vegetable prices on said "veggie-day", it could give the concept a boost and make it more attractive.

"Eat green. Drink green. Live green!", Dr. K.S. often told us, because green foods are full of energy. The energy comes from the plant pigment chlorophyll, an ingredient also abundantly found in matcha tea. Among its many health benefits, chlorophyll also has the ability to detoxify our bodies. When exposed to sunlight, the plant transforms carbon dioxides and water into carbohydrates, making it grow and flourish. Chlorophyll is practically green sunlight. And because it helps us build new blood cells, it is often known as "green blood". "Very few doctors in the western world today remember the merits of green foods", Dr. K.S. complained. Magnesium deficits are very common, which are widely due to a diet containing hardly any green vegetables while rich in fat and sugar. Without magnesium, our nervous system makes us hyper and fidgety. This mineral is vital for proper muscle activity as well as being crucial for a healthy brain.

It's a well-known fact that greens are full of important vitamins and healthy fatty acids. They are also a great source of highly effective phytonutrients. Adding a green "vegetable day" to your diet will not only benefit your health, but will also make you lose fat. Did you know that in some vegetables there are phytonutrients that, just like us, abhor abdominal fat and can attack it aggressively?

Just remember when your mom used to say: "Be sure to eat your vegetables!" That was good advice, and still valid today. Broccoli, kale, cabbage, cauliflower, Brussel sprouts, Chinese cabbage, red cabbage, kohlrabi, turnips, and beets contain unique phytonutrients that help eliminate unhealthy belly fat.

We need to incorporate fruit and vegetables in our diet to get these valuable substances into our system. Unfortunately, people often don't do this. To help melt your belly fat, follow your mom's advice and eat as many raw or cooked greens as you can.

The Brain's Appendix

I was prescribed a daily dose of 3 mg of melatonin by Dr. K.S., which I have been taking ever since. He told me to take it half an hour before going to bed, placing it under my tongue, letting the messenger substances enter my system via the mucous membranes more effectively. I had known melatonin for years because, as a frequent flyer, my husband used it for jetlag and sometimes for insomnia. But I was amazed to find out all the other wonderful things the so-called sleep hormone can do. A tiny part of the brain called the pineal gland, which produces melatonin, can make us feel younger and slow down the ageing process. Until a couple of decades ago, doctors and researchers considered this part of the brain as "useless", calling it the appendix of the brain. Recently, prominent scientists have corrected this misconception and graduated the pineal gland to being a remarkably important part of our organism. The bad news: the gland's activity starts declining during puberty. The good news: we can do something about that. Recent studies on ageing have come into focus, and discovered new correlations between the ageing process, various diseases, and melatonin levels. Melatonin is now known as a powerful antioxidant and is found in small doses in cherries, walnuts, grapes, and cocoa. Melatonin suppressors, on the other hand, are contained in coffee, nicotine, alcohol, and various medicines like beta blockers.

The melatonin our bodies produces is an antioxidant 50 times more effective than vitamin C, has no side effects and slows cell ageing. Science has yet to research the diversity of its uses in the human body.

During pregnancy, the fetus is supplied with melatonin, helping to regulate its sleep/wake cycle. After birth, if breast-fed, the baby gets natural melatonin through breast-milk. As the child grows, his pineal gland produces the hormone. The highest melatonin level is reached during childhood, and starts declining during adolescence. As we grow older, our melatonin level continuously goes down, dropping significantly around the age of 45 to 50. Around the age of 60, the pineal gland produces only half the amount it did at age 20. The ageing process has begun. And as our bodies age, so does our pineal gland, which means it is no longer able to secret as much melatonin and our susceptibility to cardio-vascular disease and cancer is increased. This drew the attention of gerontologists. They suspected these facts to be linked, and the root cause to be pineal decline and calcification, which obviously decreases melatonin secretion with age. However, the hormone's role as a messenger and regulatory substance in our body's endocrine system is extremely important. It influences our immune system, ageing process, sleep/wake cycle, mood-swings, stress awareness, sexual development, as well as our potency and libido.

Many people know melatonin only as a sleep hormone that promotes deep sleep. That is correct, since, as mentioned before, it regulates our day/night rhythm. By darkness, our retina signals our brain to produce and release melatonin, causing us to feel tired and fall into restful sleep. In daylight, melatonin secretion stops, while serotonin production is intensified; we wake up and are ready to face the challenges of the day. This is also why infants up to the age of three sleep a lot.

They produce high levels of melatonin.

Interestingly, pregnant women sleep especially well due to their melatonin level increased 300 fold.

Research on Melatonin

In the course of their research in the 1940's, Walter Pierpaoli and William Regelson, two gerontologists and melatonin experts, came across the little known pineal hormone. For over 30 years, they studied the effects of melatonin and its influence on the endocrine glandular system and gained the most astonishing new insights.

Since then, many researchers have come to the conclusion that hormone-dependent cancer such as breast or prostate cancer are caused by pineal gland deficiency. Women and men suffering from this kind of tumor, both show melatonin cycle disorders. Because their blindness causes higher levels of melatonin, blind women are far less susceptible to breast cancer.

In many studies, Pierpaoli and Regelson were able to prove that melatonin renews helper T cells. Besides their rejuvenating properties, these cells are made more aggressive towards cancer cells. Before multiplying and grouping to form a tumor, the cancer cells are detected and radically destroyed. These results are all the more stunning considering that the hormone - despite its lack of side-effects - has yet to be taken seriously within established cancer treatment. Chemotherapy, on the other hand, remains the preferred, standard therapy, even at the cost of healthy cell destruction and questionable healing rates. Melatonin proves to be very helpful in cancer prevention and cancer treatment, and it can improve quality of life while simultaneously helping to diminish the side-effects caused by chemotherapy.

Dr. Pierpaoli prescribed melatonin to his ex-mother-in-law in 1984. At the time, the woman was 74 years old and suffered from Parkinson's disease. Ten years later, she was free of all symptoms and bursting with good health and agility - even her skin was almost wrinkle-free.

INCIDENTALLY: My husband and I have both had good personal experiences with melatonin. We sleep deeply and are well-rested and in good spirits in the morning. In our personal opinion, melatonin is clearly beneficial until proven otherwise. During my own research, I found a melatonin product manufactured out of the natural ingredient cocoa. In the U.S., melatonin has been considered a miracle drug for years, and synthetic melatonin is an over-the-counter drug. A similar product has now reached Europe and Germany. However, it is a prescription drug for sleep disorders and only for people aged 55 and older.

The Arteries' Body Guard: Vitamin K

In my box of pills, there was also one jar marked "Super K". "These are good for your bones and avoiding deadly plaque, in other words, artery calcification", Dr. K.S. said. I take one of these soft-gel pills called "Super K with Advanced K2 Complex" once a day after breakfast.

The importance of the fat-soluble vitamin K for numerous functions in our system has long been established by research. It is essential for maintaining healthy bones. Also, it is a local inhibitor of calcification, by improving blood clotting and keeping calcium in the blood from binding to the arterial walls. One could almost say it works like the arteries' personal body guard. Vitamin K can prevent arteriosclerosis, which takes years to develop into degenerative damage of the vascular system, caused by the narrowing and loss of elasticity of the artery walls due to plaque buildup. The consequences can be circulation problems, thrombosis, heart attack or stroke, and the risks increase with age. Poor vitamin K status in postmenopausal women is also shown to be associated with increased bone loss, or loss of bone density. Today, research has shown that vitamin K naturally occurs in the form of vitamin K1 and K2.

Vitamin K1 is mostly found in green leafy vegetables such as red beets, broccoli, cabbage, and spinach, whereas vitamin K2 occurs in animal products like egg yolk, butter, liver, and cheese and also in the fermented soybean product known as Natto. The bacteria and microorganisms in our intestines also produce Vitamin K2. Our system can absorb vitamin K2 more easily than vitamin K1, and is also believed to be able to transform vitamin K1 into K2.

The 2004 Rotterdam Heart Study conducted for ten years on a group of 4,800 men and women aged 55 and older found that participants living on a vitamin K2-rich diet showed significantly less artery calcification than those ingesting vitamin K1. Simultaneously, the vitamin K2 group proved to have a 50 percent lower risk of dying of cardiovascular disease than the K1 group.

Because vitamin K2 absorbs directly through intestinal cells, it is especially important to have a healthy colon, since it is this organ that provides us with all the essential nutrients and trace elements we need.

An unhealthy diet and rising blood pressure leads to microscopic tears in the inner artery walls. As a result, our system tries to fix the damage by drawing on vitamin C and E. If not enough of these vital substances are available, our body compromises by patching up the fissures with a mixture of LDL cholesterol - the "bad" cholesterol - calcium and other substances in our blood. This combination in the damaged areas forms calcification buildups called plaque, which, over time, can rupture, and lead to heart attack and stroke. Vitamin K2 can reverse plaque buildup. Most people have vitamin K deficiency due to unhealthy eating and a lack of knowledge on how to avoid it. In the following is a list of foods that will help boost your vitamin K levels. Excellent sources of vitamin K are leafy green vegetables, parsley, chives, butter, egg yolk, raw sauerkraut, liver, and a variety of cheeses. Red beet leaves contain 2,000 times more vitamin K than the vegetable itself. Of all cabbage varieties, kale is the richest in vitamin K, but also cauliflower, broccoli, Brussel sprouts and white cabbage contain it. Even Sauerkraut contains vitamin K2. Avocados are not only abundant in vitamin K, but also provide the valuable fats necessary for soluble vitamin resorption.

The Truth about Eggs and Cholesterol

Perhaps some people still believe that a single egg can drastically raise their cholesterol levels. Haven't we been told for years, that eggs were guilty of this? "But that is wrong!", Dr. K.S. explained, following up with an enlightening story. He told me of his friend, who wanted to make him a hardy breakfast and, in the process of cracking half a dozen eggs, threw the egg yolks away. "Oh, my God", Dr. K.S. exclaimed. "Why are you throwing away the healthy egg yolk?", he asked his friend. "I thought the yolk was out of the question for you - it's full of nasty, bad cholesterol and fat".

He had also thrown away all the beneficial nutrients contained in the eggs. "You see, Katharina, that's the price of evil misinformation believed over the years. It only serves to make people insecure", he complained. "In reality, the yolk is the healthiest part. By comparison, the egg white holds hardly any nutrients at all. By discarding the yolk, we are throwing the most antioxidant and nutritious part down the drain." *Well, great!*

Egg yolk contains over 90 percent calcium, fat-soluble vitamin A, D and E as well as vitamin B1, B5, B6 and B12. It also contains iron, zinc, phosphorus, folic acid, lutein (double eye protection), essential fatty acids, traces of minerals and other highly valuable nutrients too numerous to list.

And worse yet is the fact that the egg white is not nearly as beneficial without (!) the egg yolk, because on its own, the protein in the egg white isn't able to balance out the amino acids.

Usually, when ingesting cholesterol-rich food such as eggs, our system can regulate a surplus. However, if we do not eat enough cholesterol necessary for a number of other important functions, our body produces its own. Many recent studies have even shown that whole eggs do not raise "good" HDL cholesterol levels any more than they do "bad" LDL cholesterol levels. In other words, the overall cholesterol ratio in our blood is improved when we eat whole eggs. Also cholesterol levels are not a disease, as opposed to osteoporosis or heart attack!

Besides lutein, egg yolk is a source of other antioxidants useful for inflammation prevention. And these inflammations are the very cause of heart disease, and not at all the cholesterol in food, which actually causes our system to reduce its own production.

In a study at the University of Connecticut, two male groups were given three eggs a day over a period of twelve weeks. The first group ate the entire egg, the second ate only the egg whites. The "egg white" group showed no change in their "good" HDL cholesterol levels. In the second group however, HDL cholesterol levels were improved, despite a reduced, but 20 percent more fatty diet, and the "bad" LDL cholesterol remained the same. This leads to the conclusion that whole eggs are not unhealthy and are much better for us than just egg whites. Also, because they are more nutritious and richer in calories, egg yolks have a higher satiation effect, thereby curbing our appetite. The healthy fat contained in egg yolk further helps keep fat-burning hormone levels balanced. This means that the substances in egg yolk support fat-burning in our system. Please bear in mind that there is no comparison to organic farm eggs, which are by far richer in nutrients than the battery cage produced eggs sold in normal supermarkets. Free-range chickens are fed naturally, which makes their eggs richer in vitamins and minerals and provides a better omega-3 to omega-6 fatty acid ratio.

A further study had one group eat scrambled eggs over a period of time, while the other group ate cereals and rolls for breakfast. The scrambled-egg group lost or held their weight, and the roll-cereal group gained weight. The assumption here is that the scrambled-egg group was less hungry during the day, and therefore had a lower calorie intake. The roll-cereal group was subject to cravings and uncontrolled blood sugar spiking. If anyone should ever tell you again that egg whites are the only valuable part of eggs, you now know better.

Reaching the Age of 100 - with Glutathione?

"Here. This little helper will slow down your ageing process.", Dr. K.S. said to me one day, pointing at one of the capsules in the big box containing the sum of my daily ration of health enhancing supplements. I was to take one a day before breakfast. Glutathione, Cysteine & C, by Life Extension. "Current statics show that centenarians are the now fastest growing age group", he continued. I wanted to know why and how. What is the secret to a long and healthy life? The answer possibly lies in a tiny, but extremely potent amino acid molecule, found in each and every cell of our bodies called glutathione. This insight is not completely new; in 1921, British biochemist and Nobel laureate Frederik Gowland Hopkins discovered the importance of glutathione for disease prevention and the sustenance of good health. Glutathione is a highly effective antioxidant with regulatory functions of various enzymatic activities in our bodies, and particularly regarding reactions impacting cancer prevention. It eliminates preformed, precursor cancer cells. Its therapeutic significance was clearly proven in a six-month study started in 2013 at Penn State College of Medicine. The extent of glutathione's role in early-stage cancer cell death is currently under examination.

Dr. K.S. says: "When treating a patient with disease-related glutathione deficiency, I administer, among other things, a high dosage of reduced glutathione to increase his or her cellular glutathione levels. As a measure in medical nutrition therapy, I recommend a diet rich in antioxidant micronutrients, in other words, eat lots of green vegetables. The same goes for large amounts of vitamin C. Unfortunately, not enough people take this advice."

Glutathione is a molecule we produce naturally and which has many crucial functions, some of which are able to support our immune system, fight inflammation and boost vital protein production. In its active form, as a so-called reduced glutathione, it can neutralize free radicals. Once it is oxidized, or used up so to speak, our system is generally able to regenerate it and bring it back to its active form. If, however, there is an overwhelming amount of free radicals, as in the case of radiation or chemotherapy, our natural glutathione is depleted and our repair system loses its reduction potential. The consequences are severe fatigue and tiredness, which is also the same problem breast cancer patients have to face for long periods of time after chemotherapy. Radiation and chemotherapy often go hand in hand with bone marrow suppression, which can be reduced with glutathione. Bone marrow suppression is given when the marrow is unable to produce sufficient red and white cells. This condition, also known as anemia, reduces patients' capacity for activity and makes them tire easily. If platelet deficiency also occurs, the patient will have a higher risk of spontaneous or excessive bleeding. Since the immune system is weakened in this case, the likelihood of severe infection is also a problem. This is where, as one of the key components of our immune system, glutathione can help. Glutathione not only participates in all detoxifying processes and the elimination of toxins such as heavy metals, but is also responsible for all protective and healing measures. Being glutathione deficient opens all doors to chronic diseases such as Crohn's disease, rheumatism, diabetes, cancer, dementia or fungal and infectious diseases. Glutathione can initiate DNA-repairing processes and neutralize free radicals. This makes it one of the most potent anti-ageing substances to help slow down premature aging of the body. It furthers production of certain types of endorphins with pain killing, mood enhancing and ant-depressant properties. Liver tissue, well-endowed with glutathione, is able to pass these substances on to the brain.

In a study comparing the glutathione levels of 41 centenarians aged between 100 and 106 with those of persons age 60 to 79, researchers found the older group to have significantly higher glutathione levels than the younger comparison group. This clearly shows a causal link between high glutathione levels and longer life expectancy. In a follow-up study, the glutathione levels of 87 women aged between 60 and 103, and all in excellent mental and physical health, were measured. Here too, the researchers found all the women's levels to be very high. This group of women was under further observation for another five years. The researchers came to the final conclusion that high levels of glutathione are characteristic in women with long life expectancy.

In one of our conversations, Dr. K.S. added: "It is possible to balance out glutathione deficits with glutathione medication. However, for the levels to be effectively, that is, actually raised, the reduced glutathione must be bio-available. If I gave, or injected a patient intravenously with purely reduced glutathione, it would rapidly react with other substances in his or her system and no longer be active. It would practically lose all positive impact. This is why therapies using "normal" reduced glutathione have no long term effects. Reduced glutathione needs to be protected from oxidation before reaching the cells. Only then should it be allowed to take on its bio-available form, to then be able to have the desired effect."

What Makes Us Sick

During another one of our appointments, Dr. K.S. fired a series of questions at me. "Aren't you wondering why some people can eat lots of rich, oily foods, dripping with fat, or fried in lard, or clarified butter and still manage to stay slim and slender? Or, how is it that others, who eat much less, maybe even sticking to low, light and diet products, and salad dressings without oil, and who only indulge in the occasional tiny snack and a little soda drink are overweight anyway?"

"Yes", was my short answer. Now I was faced with a valid question. Are fatty foods really the main cause of overweight and obesity?

Facts on Low and Light Products, Fat and Company

An Oxford University study published this year (2014) in the British medical journal, The Lancet, is very disconcerting; it reports that one third (!) of the world population is overweight or obese. In other words, 2.1 million persons are too fat. In Germany, 64 percent of all men and 49 percent of all women are affected. The study evaluated data from 188 countries, comparing them with surveys from 1980, at which time 857 million people were overweight. The scientists are especially deeply concerned about the percentage of children and adolescents affected; in Germany, one out of five children is overweight or obese.

"For 50 years, America has been disparaging coconut fat, and for 50 years now, especially in the US, not only obesity, but also cardiovascular disease is booming.", Dr. K.S. said as we broached the subject of coconut oil.

"Did the coconut take its revenge for this?", I responded spontaneously. Here in South East Asia, everyone fries their food with oil in woks. They use massive amounts of clarified butter, which is very popular and known as ghee. According to international studies, the world-famous Mediterranean diet, in which vegetables are prepared with olive oil and served with fatty lamb is responsible for one of the highest life expectancies. For generations, the inhabitants of the remote South East Asian islands and archipelagos have been consuming coconut oil. And despite that, hardly any of them suffer from overweight. "For years, it was repeatedly propagated that cooking fat was to be avoided. Anyone voicing a different opinion got in trouble with non-other than the DGE - the German Nutrition Society. The mistake that was made and which everyone has now internalized over the years, is the indiscriminate claim, that fat makes you fat, and consuming it is unhealthy.", said certified agricultural engineer Stefanie Goldscheider of the online magazine for nutrition and agriculture Biothemen.de in an email to me. But, fat is actually undeserving of its bad reputation. The truth is, fat is essential for our survival and we need it! Without it, our bodies are incapable of absorbing certain important vitamins, just as our cells cannot function without it. However, everything depends on *which* fats we ingest. As a rule of thumb, the softer and more liquid a fat is, the more unsaturated fatty acids it contains. These unsaturated fats are much better for our systems than the saturated ones. And although we are not naturally able to produce unsaturated fats, we can draw them from plant fats.

The widespread assumption that all vegetable fats are beneficial, and all animal fats are harmful is not scientifically tenable. The human body actually needs both types. In other words, animal and vegetable fat in combination are vital. For example, two tablespoons of vegetable fat (unsaturated) and a little butter (saturated) make a good combination. So far so good.

Meat and butter contain saturated fats, and also a lot of cholesterol. Normally, a healthy body can easily process this and maintain its balance. However, when faced with an excess of saturated fats, as is often the case in our modern-day foods, our cholesterol levels can be thrown out of balance. This is exactly what causes high risk of heart attack and stroke. A healthy body should show higher levels of HDL cholesterol, and lower levels of LDL cholesterol. Why? For the simple reason that the "bad" LDL cholesterol is the cholesterol delivering agent, enabling cells to function properly. The "good" HDL cholesterol is the cleaning crew, so to speak, responsible for collecting excess fat in the blood. If too much LDL is delivered, our blood gets overwhelmed by a surplus of saturated fatty acids. The so-called cleaning crew is then no longer able to handle the excess fats, and cholesterol builds up on the inner arterial walls. As the fat deposits grow, they block the blood flow and if, in a worst case scenario, one of these deposits is near the heart, it is likely to cause a heart attack. Similar problems can also be caused by the use of cholesterol lowering margarine, due to high levels of added plant sterols, which contain fat-like substances. These sterols are a kind of plant cholesterol found in fruit and vegetables. Vegetable oils made of sunflowers seeds, soy beans, wheat germ, and nuts are abundant in plant sterols. Generally, 0.07oz per day is enough to lower elevated cholesterol levels. However, German Federal Institute for Risk Assessment studies found that cholesterol lowering margarines also contain extremely high concentrations of plant sterols which have very little to do with natural nutrition and are even considered to be hazardous to our health. The "overdose" increases the risk of heart attack and stroke to an extremely high rate. The same can be said for all products labeled "low", "light", "bio", and "active", and those claiming to be cholesterol lowering.

"But why then, did the healthy coconut oil disappear?", I asked Dr. K.S. Etiologists believe the powerful agricultural lobby is to blame. Their main goal is to promote their own products. Coconut oil, which was popular until then, and which I remember my mother cooking and baking with, finally disappeared into oblivion. In contrast, industrially produced margarine was presented worldwide as the ideal solution, and soon "low fat" and "light" products flooded the market as well. Simultaneously, fast-food burger chains became famous all over the globe, leaving local products from poorer countries behind. The food-oil industry refined oil, and the healthier product disappeared.

"In any case", Dr. K.S. finally said, "the truth is, that despite fat contents decreasing in low and light food products over the past 30 years, people are still getting fatter and fatter." Processed foods of all kinds, sweets, pastries, and all deep-fried foods have little or nothing to do with natural foods, which are prepared with animal fats or organic and carefully pressed vegetable oils. And what's worse, according to our Doc, is that trans fats are not only a by-product of industrial fat hardening, but also occur through cooking with these oils at high temperatures. Trans fats are the real evildoers making us sick and fat.

"Could artificial fats, similar in taste and consistency, due to various fat substitutes to make them seem like authentic fats, stimulate cravings, the way artificial sweeteners do?" I asked Dr. K.S. "That could very well be possible. The fact remains, that low-calorie, sugar-free, fat-reduced, and low, light, and diet food products do not contribute to weight loss. Nor do artificial, cholesterol lowering products lead to lower cholesterol levels. Diseases like obesity, diabetes, heart attack, stroke, cancer and arteriosclerosis are constantly on the rise. If people do not see the truth about all this and do not change their way of thinking about food and alter their nutritional habits, we are headed for disaster!" Natural fats are crucial for our nerves, brain, for all our membranes, and our entire hormone balance. Cooking with coconut oil or ingesting just one tablespoon per day will set you on the right path. In any case, I can guarantee, that your steak, chicken, baking, vegetables, and much more will provide you with a brand-new culinary sensation. With this natural, healthy oil, we can even enjoy French-fries, potato chips, pastries, and other delicacies without any remorse.

INCIDENTALLY: Regardless of all concerns, humans need fat! On a daily basis, our bodies need to renew and repair approximately 50 million cells. For this to function properly, we need about 0.0175oz of fat per pound of body weight. A person weighing about 132 pounds should consume 2.11oz of fat. A healthy combination would consist of ghee (animal fat) and coconut oil (vegetable fat). Also other types of cold pressed vegetable oils are suitable, provided they are not over-heated. We need animal fat to metabolize carbohydrates, ensuring the slow transformation of carbohydrates into energy. This means that our breakfast can be rich in carbohydrates. With bread, rolls (no wheat!, no gluten!), potatoes and eggs (fried in coconut oil or cooked), it is the heartiest meal of the day. Also, sweet homemade jam with healthy bread. For lunch, we are allowed to eat almost anything we want – except fast food, in plastic packaged and already finished cooked food! Dinner should be rich in protein, consisting of meat or fish and vegetables. Cold cuts and cheese are also permitted. Please do not eat too much high-fat cheese. A good rule to follow is: no carbohydrates after 4:00 pm, which also includes fruit, fruit juice and raw(!) vegetables and no(!) salad.

Attention Calorie Counters!

We tend to believe that we lose weight if our food is low in calories, and vice-versa. This is incorrect. Although the total amount of calories ingested in relation to the number of calories burned is an important aspect in weight loss, many more factors play a roll, considering that hardly anyone is able to count calories accurately. According to various studies, 75 to 90 percent of people counting their calories misjudge their intake, making calorie-counting diets not really useful. Did you know that one of our most important fat-burner hormones is reduced when we go on a diet of this kind? Researchers at the Munich Helmholtz Center found that two hormones stimulate fat metabolism and regulate our weight. In the future, they could be a serious weapon in the battle against overweight and obesity. One of them is glucagon, working in tandem with insulin, but with the opposite effect. Glucagon causes glucose to be released when our blood sugar levels are low, and activates an enzyme to transform fat into energy. The second hormone is FGF21. Also produced by the liver, it boosts fat metabolism. Studies on mice were done to observe the hormones' long-term effects. The mice that were given glucagon ate less, while simultaneously showing an increase in fat-burning, but their cholesterol levels decreased, while secreting significantly more FGF21. The same effect was observed in humans. Glucagon has an impressive ability to make fat deposits melt away. After just seven days of dieting, the glucagon hormone level shrinks by up to 50 percent. In other words, the longer we are on this kind of "normal" diet, the worse our health gets. That is why people on constant diets are in a permanent battle with their weight control.

When we eat the wrong foods, our hormone balance is disrupted, which can lead to over-eating. Our metabolism gets sluggish and further problems arise, preventing effective weight loss. However, by eating the right and healthy foods, we can stimulate our metabolism and turn our bodies into virtual "fat-burning machines".

Unfortunately, the so-called food pyramid is misleading, and the deceptive, and sometimes fraudulent labels of various food producers send our efforts to lose fat down the wrong path. Many food products advertised as healthy or especially slimming are the very ones that make us put on even more fat. Among these, are apple and orange juice, soy milk, skim milk, energy drinks like "Gatorade" and other industrially manufactured sports drinks, protein bars, diet ice-cream and desserts, low-fat foods, low-carb foods (based on consistent omission of any carbs), soy oil, corn oil, and rapeseed oil (please never use this one ever again!). Also on the list are whole-grain breads, whole-grain cereals and crackers, burgers in all varieties, tofu, veggie burgers, margarine, rice cakes, and pasta. All these foods cause cravings and sabotage our constant efforts to lose fat. And worst of all is the fact that they throw our hormone balance off kilter.

Beware of Harmful Fats!

The debate on which cooking oils are harmful and which are not is still on-going. In 2001, canola oil, or rapeseed oil, appeared on the market, and claimed to be the healthiest cooking oil of all times. But, be careful! The exact opposite is true. You will be shocked to learn the facts on its actual effects on human health, which were published in the Wall Street Journal as early as 1995.

141

Rapeseed oil seeds have been used for industrial purposes for a long time, and are poisonous for humans and animals alike. The seeds are used as a substance to illuminate the colors of glossy magazine pages, and also as biodiesel, as a synthetic rubber base, and as solvents, surfactants (detergents) and lubricants.

Rapeseed oil is an industrial product, appropriate for industrial use only and is not a food! It can cause emphysema, which are abnormal over-inflation of cavity organs such as the lung, resulting in shortness of breath, blindness, anemia and irritability.

A further fact of particular interest that everyone should consider is that the sheep disease, scrapie, which humans suffer from in the form of Creutzfeldt-Jakob, and cattle contract as mad cow disease, disappeared once rapeseeds were removed from sheep feed. Animal meal stemming from infected sheep had been fed to cattle, thereby transferring the pathogens and causing the outbreak of mad cow disease. Once the cause was determined, rapeseed was no longer added to the animal meal and, not surprisingly, since then, no further cases of mad cow disease have been reported.

Despite all this, the food industry still uses rapeseeds in thousands of processed foods. They go so far as to claim that "rapeseed oil is completely safe, because, thanks to genetic modification (!), we are no longer dealing with rapeseeds as such, but with canola." Although they do admit that canola is a rapeseed product. So, by simply changing the name, the substance changes?! No matter how rapeseeds may have been modified, they are still part of the rape plant.

Studies on lab animals, that were given canola oil, produced devastating results.

If you wish to avoid oil that can make you sick, and especially genetically modified foods, the best thing to do is cross rapeseed oil and canola off your shopping list for good! Unless you need it to free the roses in your garden from pests. Rapeseed oil is an excellent pesticide against aphids. Or you can use it on your squeaky doors. "But please, never use rapeseed oil as a food again!", says Dr. K.S.

Health Risk: Trans Fats

As I described at length earlier, some cooking oils, such as my favorite, coconut oil, are very healthy, whereas others, like rapeseed oil, are extremely detrimental to our health. Unfortunately, there are other oils equally bad for us, especially when used for pan and deep-frying, due to the unhealthy trans fats the process generates. Dr. K.S. quotes nutrition expert and Harvard University Professor Walter Willet, who saw the dangers of trans fats years ago: "They're doubly dangerous because they elevate the 'bad' LDL, while lowering the 'good' HDL cholesterol levels in our blood. This increases the risk of inflammation and the dangers for our arteries. It leads to heart attack, stroke and other terrible diseases."

Not only the oil manufacturing process itself is a source of hazardous trans fats, but also cooking and frying with sunflower oil, soybean oil, corn, thistle and olive oil - high temperatures transforms their unsaturated components into dangerous trans fats. These are found in most of our food today - in all deep fried foods like French fries, German curry sausages, fish sticks, chicken wings, and potato chips. Also pastries such as jelly donuts, croissants, puff pastry and processed foods like spreads, powdered gravies and soups, processed meats, breakfast cereals and granola bars all contain trans fats.

In 2006, the alarming news about trans fats hit New York, causing great concern among nutrition experts and medical doctors. Even though it was well known at the time that these fatty acids were damaging to the heart and arteries, hardly any restaurants, fast food places, cafés or donut bakeries stopped using the unsafe fats. In 2008, a law forbidding the use of trans fats in food products was issued to protect hundreds of thousands of people from heart disease. This measure was received with great turbulence by the U.S. media, who saw the nearing end of our treasured French-fries, also especially because Chicago was also willing to ban trans fats. Since then, many restaurants and kitchens in the U.S. have switched to different oils such as sunflower and sesame oil. The disaster, however, is still not under control because as soon as these oils are overheated, for example for deep frying, consumers still ingest trans fats.

The danger trans fats poses was understood not only in the United States. In 2003, Denmark, as the sole European Union pioneer in matters regarding trans fats, issued the following restrictions: All food products on the market are to be limited to a maximum of two percent trans fats. The same applies to imported products. Similar regulations were passed in Austria in 2009, and since 2011, in California, there is a complete ban on the dangerous fats.

However, Germany, and the remaining European Union, has not yet followed suit with restricting - not to mention banning - the fats! According to the EU Food Information Regulation, it is against the law to mention trans fats on food labels. Excuse me? you might ask. The German Nutrition Society, DGE, merely recommends keeping food energy in the form of trans fats to a minimum of one percent (as of 2012). How in the world is the consumer supposed to know what percentage of trans fats he or she is actually pouring into his or her system on a daily basis? Is there a measuring device available for that? In Austria, children especially were found to be consuming up to 0.211oz. per day. A bag of fries, please, a box of cookies, a couple of Danish at the bakery, in between a big bag of chips, to finish, a curry wurst (German hot dog with curry and ketchup sauce) and the limit is reached. In fact, the maximum allowed for adults has been surpassed. Fast-food consuming kids today have an extremely frightening intake of dangerous trans fatty acids. As shown in a study across 20 countries, they consume 20 grams (0.705oz.) of trans fats with every meal!

If these "killer fats" are proven to be the cause not only of overweight but also of inflammations leading to severe diseases such as heart attack, stroke, diabetes, and cancer, I personally do not want a single percent of them in my food, or in my body. But if producers continue to avoid proper labelling because of bad publicity, there is little or nothing we can do to escape the killer fats. This is insane! For example, peanut oil contains 35 percent trans fatty acids!

Really, the only oil stable enough to withstand high temperatures while searing or frying without generating trans fats is cold pressed coconut oil! So, before buying that Danish at the baker's, you might want to ask yourself in which fat this delicacy was fried or baked.

A Detrimental Imbalance

A further health danger Dr. K.S. was keen to draw our attention to is found in the many types of vegetable oils capable of disrupting our omega-3 versus omega-6 fatty acid balance. And we find these oils - often labeled as "healthy" in every supermarket. An omega-3 - omega-6 fatty acid imbalance also causes inflammations in our system, leading to an array of diseases. A worldwide comparison showed a clear link between heart attack and stroke and an omega-3 - omega-6 imbalance.

Recent findings were able to prove that this discrepancy had a higher health impact than unhealthy cholesterol levels.

Most people in Germany and other countries around the world live on diets with an unhealthy omega-6 to omega-3 ratio.

Ideally, the ratio should be between 1:1 and 3:1. In other words, we should be ingesting as many omega-3 as we are omega-6 fatty acids, but not more than three times as many omega-6 fatty acids. Yet in Germany, the proportion lies between 10:1 and 50:1(!). The German Nutrition Society has a different view on this, recommending a ratio of 5:1, and published a statement saying: "The current fatty acid ratio in Germany is 8:1 or 7:1." Be this as it may, our ancestors lived on food with an essential omega-6 to omega-3 ratio between 1:1 and 2:1.

The imbalance in the United States, as in Germany, Switzerland, and Austria is alarming. The reason for this is not only because we eat less fish than the Japanese, Inuits and Greenlanders, (who, by the way, have a mortality rate, due to cardio-vascular disease, of twelve percent as opposed to forty percent in Germany) but also because our animal products today contain much less omega-3 fatty acids than in former times. In the past, livestock were free-range, grazing farm animals; today most are held in narrow stalls and fed on processed grain and soy, which is more economical than other feeds, more efficient and enhances faster growth. However, these animals lack the omega-3 of green fodder. The same can be said of farmed fish.

Further reasons for this imbalance are environmental influences and our daily consumption of packaged, processed foods such as salad dressings, farmed fish, milk products, and mayonnaise. But also grain products like bread or pasta, cornflakes, cake, pastries, waffles, crackers, pretzel sticks and so on. Not all grain products should be discarded completely, but their omega-6 fatty acid content is usually predominant. As an example: rye has between 11:1 and 5:1; wheat: 14:1; corn: 29:1; and soy: from 10:1 to 5:1. I find this all very alarming.

Consuming meat, as well as meat and milk products from factory farms only aggravates the problem, by leading to an excess of omega-6 fatty acids in our system.

An equally important aspect is the growing use of artificial omega-6 fatty acids, added to cooking oils and industrial margarine. For decades, overblown advertising has promoted essential fatty acids, without distinguishing the significant differences between the two types of fatty acids. Common margarine contains 82 times (!) more omega-6 than omega-3 fatty acids. Sunflower oil has a ratio of 122:1 and thistle oil's proportions are 148:1!

These oils are practically everywhere - in processed and deep-fried foods, in baked as in pan-fried foods. We are basically being overfed and fattened by all these omega-6 rich foods.

Meanwhile, in extreme contrast, the omega-3 fatty acid content in our nutrition is being drastically reduced. Because we are creatures of habit, the fast food industry prays on us by supporting our dependencies. Today, we know that the addictive, taste-enhancing substances added in fast food can make us lose control over our eating behavior. This causes us to miss out on the foods rich in vital omega-3 fatty acids such as vegetables, lettuce, sprouts, flaxseed oil, walnuts, mushrooms, venison and fish, green algae, and wild plants and herbs. Meat, milk and cheese from free-range animals offer three to four times the amount of omega-3 fatty acids than the same products from their incarcerated cousins. The more green fodder the animals are fed, the higher the omega-3 content. The same is true of poultry fed with flaxseed, which, as an oil, is also an excellent source of omega-3. But the prime source is chia seeds, by far exceeding all others with its capacity to provide an optimal omega-3 - omega-6 balance in our bodies.

So, what is this whole imbalance really about? Again, Dr. K.S. gave us the illuminating explanation. An excess of omega-6 fatty acids stimulates inflammation causing molecules, known as eicosanoids in medical terms. These are a product of metabolized, unsaturated fatty acids, which, much like a small, steadily burning fire, attack healthy cells. Our system is thereby put into a constant state of defense, causing it to constrict the arteries, and slow down the flow of blood. This disruption of vital blood circulation eventually damages the heart. According to leading medical professors, these inflammations caused by an omega-3 - omega-6 fatty acid imbalance are the main cause for a worldwide increase in joint pain, sluggish metabolism, heart disease, weight gain, rapid ageing, skin disorders, mood swings, sugar cravings and deteriorating memory function.

If you wish to bring your omega-3 - omega-6 ratio back into balance, I recommend taking the following off your diet plan: all ready-made meals, microwave-dinners and the like, farmed fish, meat from factory farming, industrially produced milk and milk products, and non-organic eggs from battery farming. Take two to three tablespoons of chia seeds a day. This superfood is abundant in omega-3 fatty acids and shows an omega-3 to omega-6 fatty acid ratio of 3:1. And more importantly, please stop using all the "bad" cooking oils mentioned above. These oils are often loaded with omega-6 fatty acids. Another way to get your balance back would be to eat omega-3 rich fatty fish, crustaceans, and seafood.

To change our ratio from the typical 20:1 back to 1:1, we would have to ingest huge amounts of seafood and crustaceans. However, eating four pounds of shrimp, or fatty fish like wild tuna and salmon on a daily basis is not everyone's cup of tea.

Another problem is that wild seafood is not easily obtained, since most fish for sale is farm raised, which contains far more inflammatory omega-6 fatty acids than wild fish. Testing of three types of fish showed significantly higher contents of omega-6 fats than in wild fish. To make matters worse, farmed fish are mass treated with anti-biotics and more exposed to concentrated pesticides than their cousins in the wild. Industrial salmon farms use artificial color to make the farmed fish - whose flesh is typically grayish white - appear a more appetizing "salmon" pink.

"But can't I just take fish oil capsules to balance my fatty-acid ratio?", I asked Dr. K.S., in an attempt to interrupt his lecture. "There are many more important factors at play here", he replied instantly. "Fish oil contains not only omega-3 fats, but also large amounts of omega-6 fatty acids, which means we are ingesting a lot of omega fatty acids, yet are not changing the omega-3 - omega-6 ratio. Additionally, fish oil tends to be strongly contaminated with heavy metals and other harmful substances. So, omega-3 capsules are not really a good alternative and which, in an overdose, can actually lead to health problems. Due to a lack of natural antioxidants, fish oil is not stable. It quickly becomes rancid and inedible, even causing unpleasant, fish-smelling burping." "But if fish oil is not the solution either, then what is?", I asked. And once again, he reminded me of the Antarctic, shrimp-like, tiny crustaceans, which are a part of plankton, and populate the South Polar Seas in endless swarms, called krill (see page 113).

Of Milk and Men

"Every day, my grandmother gave us three kids home-made milk", Dr. K.S. was telling me during one of our talks. Home-made milk? "Yes, made of almonds." He went on to explain why I (and everybody else) should stop drinking milk. "Do you have any idea of what milk actually contains?", he asked, showing me a photo.

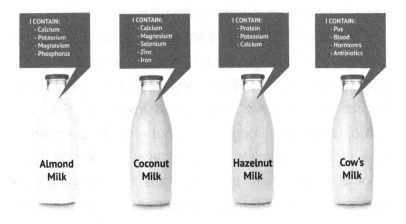

Cow milk contains millions of pus cells, as well as numerous blood segments, anti-biotics, growth hormones, and causes osteoporosis. Cow udders are sensitive, are easily infected and are never clinically clean. This causes the cows emotional and physical suffering. Cow milk is naturally meant only for their calves. If you read and understand this, you will no longer need to drink milk from another creature's milk glands! Thankfully, according to my blood-type, cow milk is a no-go and never having liked milk much, even as a child,

I had no problem skipping cow milk. But his devastating viewpoint on milk was disquieting. Even our alternative healthcare practitioner in Berlin asked my husband years ago: "Why do you drink milk? Are you a cow?"

An increasing number of scientists confirm that milk is not at all healthy, and furthermore, makes us sick. The German Nutrition Society recently found that approximately 15 percent of all adults suffer from lactose intolerance. The body is no longer able to split the naturally occurring lactose, or milk sugar, and will experience diarrhea, nausea, lots of gas, and stomach aches.

With alarming regularity, milk is found to contain environmental pollutants, heavy metals, antibiotics, pus, and blood. Osteoporosis is on the rise in countries with high milk consumption. This animal protein causes calcium drain. If calves were fed the milk we buy in supermarkets, they would die within weeks.

The so-called China Study, which caused a worldwide stir, linked the consumption of milk products to various types of cancer, such as ovarian cancer. It strongly suggested a correlation between high occurrences of growth factors similar to insulin, known as IGF-I, and prostate and breast cancer. People with regular milk product intake are found to have high counts of IGF-I in their blood. Men with equally high amounts of it in their blood are exposed to four times (!) the risk of developing prostate cancer.

Other substances found in cow milk increase insulin-like growth factors. Harvard University conducted a study on 75,000 women over a period of twelve years, to test the effects of milk on their bones. The conclusion was, that milk does not strengthen bone stability, on the contrary, the study found a connection between increased risk of bone fracture and milk consumption. Dr. K.S. and other doctors explain this with the body's hyperacidity caused by drinking milk. To neutralize the acidity, our body uses the calcium stored in our bones, thereby causing osteoporosis.

Scientists in Vietnam examined the bone substance of 105 Buddhist nuns, aged between 50 and 85, and living on a strictly vegan diet. Their bones were flawless and perfectly healthy. A healthy diet, with lots of vegetables can improve bone density. Broccoli, Brussel sprouts and various lettuces contain between 40 to 50 percent calcium. The good news for those of us who dislike eating large amounts of vegetables is that calcium can also be found in hard cheeses, preferably sheep and goat cheeses of organic quality. Also organic yoghurt, besides being a great source of protein, is rich in calcium. I just recently discovered goat's milk yoghurt.

Another excellent alternative to cow milk is milk made of almonds, quinoa, oats, and rice. Almond milk is even much more than just an alternative, since it is suitable for people with lactose intolerance. Except, of course, for people with an almond allergy. The variety of possible uses of nut-milk is endless. Any recipe using cow milk, can be adjusted by replacing it with nut milk, such as in coffee beverages like latte and cappuccino; muesli, dessert creams, pudding, cake, ice cream and much more.

In time, making almond milk from scratch myself, I became increasingly creative. And my personal best is coconut-almond milk.

Incidentally, almonds are the only alkaline nut variety. They are rich in unsaturated fatty acids, provitamin A, vitamin B and C, enzymes, calcium, potassium, magnesium, iron, carbohydrates and protein. You can make milk out of almost all nuts: cashews, walnuts, Brazil nuts, peanuts and coconuts.

Despite the controversy on cow milk, one thing is sure, the majority of people worldwide cannot drink it due to the missing lactase enzyme, necessary to digest milk sugar or lactose, which causes gas and diarrhea. For centuries, Traditional Chinese Medicine has been critical of cow milk as being mucous generating and labeled it with the attributes "cold and wet". Many parents of asthmatic children agree and are even convinced that cow milk worsens the symptoms. Meanwhile, many doctors today are advising patients suffering from colds or chronic sinus infections to give up cow milk altogether. Symptoms generally disappear within days. Experts especially recommend avoiding cow milk in case of inflammatory rheumatic disease.

Nutritionist Christina Alder, specialized in patient training at the Swiss League Against Rheumatism, sees this quite differently. "This is a delicate subject. Despite a lot of practical knowledge, there's still too little systematic research." Excuse me? Doesn't practical knowledge count for anything? This knowledge comes from the experience of affected people! Having personally suffered from rheumatism (!) so extremely, I was hardly able to move anymore, I strongly advise you to avoid cow milk. The inflammatory substance contained in cow milk and cream is known as arachidonic acid.

I recommend choosing healthier alternatives. Not only can you make your own "milk" from scratch, but also your own almond butter.

Further Milk Alternatives

- Grain milk is lactose-free. But its nutritional value regarding vitamins and minerals certainly matches that of cow milk. This milk is made mainly of rye, oats and spelt, yet contains less protein.
- Goat, sheep and mare's milk are ideal alternatives for people with allergies to whey protein contained in cow milk. However, goat milk is not suitable in case of lactose intolerance, due to the similar content of lactose.
- Rice milk is generally made of brown rice, supplemented with vitamins and calcium to make

up for a lack of nutritional components. Its protein content lies between 0.1 and 0.3 percent. Rice milk, is a better alternative because, as opposed to soy milk, it contains less allergens.

A Healthy Gut is Key to Overall Good Health

Clearly, all of Dr. K.S.'s wonderful advice that I've shared with you, and will continue to elaborate upon, makes little sense if your gut is compromised and not healed before a dietary change. Remember Paracelsus, whom I quoted at the beginning of this book, saying: "Death resides in the intestines!" Greek physician Hippocrates, phrasing it not quite as drastically, said: "A healthy gut is the source of all good health". This is why Dr. K.S.'s 7-day detox plan is essential, to bring our gut back to functioning at its best, to be able to metabolize the vital substances and enzymes in our food. This will not succeed with a clogged gut!

Some people do not understand the meaning of colon cleansing. What is there to cleanse? Is there even anything in there that needs cleansing? Makes no sense…

I think everyone is entitled to their own opinion. However, what is undeniable, is the fact that the major part of our immune system is located in our bowels. As our largest organ, the intestine can reach a length of 26ft. and a surface of 5,381.9 sq. ft. Viewed from this angle, I do think that cleansing over 5,000 sq. ft. of our bodies sounds worthwhile. The thought of climbing into a sewer pipe draining tons of feces on a daily basis is not exactly appetizing, is it? And, if we consider the fact that a single human being eliminates about 50 liters of stool per year and around 500 liters of urine, we get a pretty good picture of what goes on in our bowels over the years. In the course of a lifetime, tons of food and tens of thousands of liters of liquid are passed through our intestines. And of course, countless pathogenic germs and toxins travel right along, making this a huge processing task. We know now, that not everything can be eliminated and that some of it gets stuck for a long time in the many windings of the intestine. Not a great thing to visualize either, right? It's as though we mopped the floor without ever getting into the corners. Today, doctors know that diverticulosis, among other diseases, can be caused by polluted intestines. According to a 2010 study, 16 percent of men and 14 percent of women in Germany were suffering from this disease, which causes pouches, called diverticula, to form in the wall of both the small and the large intestine. When several of these pouches are aligned in the intestinal wall, the condition is called diverticulosis. After decades of pressure, caused by constipation or gas, the wall tissue, especially in the large intestine, tends to get worn out and lose its firmness. The more pressure there is on the wall and more the tissue weakens, and the faster these small pouches or blisters called diverticula will form.

They can reach a length of almost 2 inches! The bad thing though, is that stool almost always collects in them. These waste remains cause toxic depots in our system as well as forming pellet-like hard stools. Some doctors say that people not yet suffering from the condition are very likely to contract it at some point because it is as common as losing hair, and the likelihood of developing this condition increases dramatically with age. Although generally not life-endangering, the disease can have serious consequences if the diverticula are inflamed. In some cases, only surgical removal of the affected colon area can help.

Diverticulosis is definitely a by-product of our highly civilized life-style. The disease occurs far more rarely in third world countries. In view of this fact, we should ask ourselves, what are we doing wrong? We don't want to change our comfortable life-style, giving up our dish washers, nice cars, beautiful homes, and yearly vacations. And we don't have to. But, regarding our diets, we should urgently give our life-style some serious thought.

Diverticulosis has recently developed into an epidemic. The reason for this is that we eat too much of too many unhealthy foods, too quickly, and too late in the day. A diet rich in fibers, relatively low on carbohydrates, and with lots of vegetables has shown excellent results in the battle against this disease.

The gut goes to bed and rises with the chickens, as the saying goes. This means the healthiest way to eat is before 6:00 PM. Dr. K.S. explained, "Our organ clock as well as Chinese Medicine have both proven that to recuperate, our intestines take a break for approximately twelve hours. During this time, our bodies are working full steam to make us fit for the next day. At night, food lingers in our digestive system, that is, in our stomach and small and large intestines. And because the food is not digested properly, toxins are easily formed." We often notice this through an odd taste in our mouths and a coated tongue the morning after an elaborate barbeque party or lavish celebration. Instead, in the evening we should be eating small portions of lighter food.

Most people know the saying: "Eat breakfast like a king, lunch like a prince, and dinner like a pauper". Yet for many, due to their work schedules, dinner has become the main meal. In Mediterranean countries, people are accustomed to eating late in the evening, but hardly eat anything for breakfast. Their first substantial meal is often not before noon, leaving the system enough time to digest.

We, on the other hand, have breakfast as early as 6:00 or 7:00 AM, and often have to hurry to get to school or the office on time.

Some years ago, a friend and colleague of mine, Jürgen Schilling, wrote a book about the consequences of eating too quickly called "Healthy Chewing". Having developed this method of eating slowly 23 years ago, he was able to overcome a chronic, supposedly incurable gastro-intestinal disease. And, incidentally, without depriving himself in the least, he managed to lose over 72 lbs. Jürgen Schilling coined the expression "Jaw Jogging", to describe slow chewing, while savoring without hasty gulping. Today his work-shops are subsidized by national health insurance companies. A study shows that, as opposed to normal chewing, "jaw jogging" prevents blood sugar levels from rising, or barely rising at all. This way the insulin production is curbed and the risk of diabetes significantly reduced. Among scientists, insulin is also known as the "hunger hormone", based on the fact that almost all overweight people suffer from metabolic imbalance. Their bodies produce too much insulin, which triggers hunger.

Not only do we eat too much, too much unhealthy food, and we also throw too much of it away too quickly. Even honey has to be labeled with an expiration date these days - an absurd bureaucratic regulation, since 3,000-year-old honey was discovered in pharaoh tombs and found to be perfectly edible today.

It goes without saying, that we obviously shouldn't eat spoiled foods.

What Goes on in the Gut

In answer to my question on what exactly the intestine's job is, Dr. K.S. drew another deep breath and jumped into a long lecture. In his opinion, not only stress makes us sick, but mostly an unhealthy, compromised gut.

Our stomach breaks down our daily food and blends it. Eventually, this blend is passed on to the small intestine for further processing. At this stage, the nutrients contained in the food are released and metabolized. However, compromised intestines burdened with deposits, putrid waste, and fermentation are the perfect breeding ground for health problems and numerous diseases. The main culprit here are protein-rich foods, which, in combination with fat and carbohydrates are mucus-forming. The worst offenders are fatty dairy products, grains in excess, especially wheat products, animal protein, and processed meat, and all varieties of candy and sweets.

Once the gut is thoroughly encrusted, now all you need in the mix to destroy the intestinal flora are preservatives, chlorinated drinking water, alcoholic beverages, nicotine, medicine - especially antibiotics. Now lots of space is cleared for all kinds of microforms to take over, such as harmful fungus, putrid bacteria, worms and intestinal fluke. Fermentation begins in the gut, producing liver damaging ethanol, and at your next check-up, the doctor finds bad liver function results and tells you to check your alcohol consumption.

The author of this book, ergo yours truly, strongly recommends changing your nutrition to improve your health, because I am living proof of the sensational results.

However, is eating healthy foods, rich in fiber, and taking all the right supplements enough to be healthy again? Unfortunately, not in all cases! If our gut lining is no longer able to absorb most of the essential vital nutrients, this causes nutritional deficiencies in our cells. And even if we are eating healthy foods, we still suffer from deficiency caused diseases. How can this be? The answer is simple. After years of unhealthy eating, our intestinal walls are thickly coated with slimy, sticky and sometimes hardened stool masses. All the wonderfully healthy foods now rot and ferment, contributing to our further toxicity, to make matters worse. Well done!

So, without healing our gut, no amount of healthy, fiber-rich food will do us any good.

In answer to those critical of colon cleansing - and there are many - I ask, do we not brush our teeth every day, because dentists warn us that not doing so regularly is bad for us? New Zealand dentists were able to prove that keeping your teeth clean can prolong your life by seven years, because patients free of periodontal disease and mouth inflammation live 6.4 years longer in average, thanks to their lower risk of cardio-vascular disease and diabetes.

Food actually stays in the mouth for a limited length of time, and food remains are eliminated fairly quickly through dental hygiene. However, by comparison, it can take up to three days for the chewed up food masses to be excreted. That being the case, we can only imagine the terrible condition our gut must be in.

Why do we wash our car before applying polish to make it shiny? I doubt you would put polish onto the dirty surface of your car, and then rub it to a polish. So why should we take better loving care of our household items than of our gut, which is the largest organ in our body?

Many people are unhappy with the results of a weight-loss diet and complain that nothing much has changed. But how could it? When giving a wood framed window a new coat of paint, doesn't the painter start by sanding down the old paint to allow the pores in the wood to open up and breath, so the new paint can adhere properly?

Clearly, this shows that a colon cleanse every now and then makes absolute sense. As for those substances our bodies may need, but which were eliminated in the cleansing process, these are easily replaced through a healthy and varied diet.

70 percent of the immune cells our intestines produce live inside the gut itself. The gut flora, which consists of billions of microorganisms, mainly produces lactobacilli, which in turn produce important essential vitamins such as vitamin A and K, along with folic acid, which are involved in all growth and developing processes in our body. Normally, our intestines are perfectly able to balance out short-term strains without our even noticing. Long-term and serious over-burdening however, will destabilize the flora balance considerably. When this

happens, we face negative effects on our entire immune system.

On Acids and Bases

Would you have thought there was a connection between having cellulite and hyperacidity? Because this problem is caused by an acid-base imbalance, Dr. K.S. combined the blood-type diet with a balanced acid-base diet. He is certain that the acid-base balance plays an essential role in our overall health and well-being. It is therefore important to have a balanced "household", without which we can develop severe illnesses over a period of many years. Perfect equilibrium ensures hormone balance, well-functioning digestion, healthy breathing, stable circulation, a strong immune system and facilitates elimination of toxic waste from our system. Unfortunately, environmental changes as well as our modern-day dietary habits and life-styles often upset this balance.

I Will Not Be Sour Anymore

Hyperacidity in our body comes from acid-forming and acidic foods like fast foods, low-alkaline food products, trans fats, diabetes type 2, as well as nicotine, stress, digestive disorders and much more. For all the processes in our system to function at their best, the pH in our blood and inside our cells should lie between 7.35 and 7.45. Our body is constantly working to maintain these levels. To keep the vital pH levels at an optimal balance in our blood, our body has several ways of dealing with excess acidity. One is to excrete it via the skin, the kidneys and the intestine, another way is through the so-called buffer system. While our connective tissues, joints and muscles serve as acid depots, our buffer system normally balances out sudden excess acidity in the blood by releasing neutralizing alkaline substances. However, capacity for acid storage is limited. Once this limit is reached and no further acid can be stored or neutralized, certain vital functions are disrupted and endangered. We feel discomfort, muscle tension, fatigue, back and neck pain, suffer from skin disorders, cellulite, vital substance deficiency, or even chronic diseases such as gout, osteoporosis, polyarthritis and chronic acidosis. The acid forming substances are chlorine, sulfur and phosphorus. Their natural alkaline forming counterparts are magnesium, sodium, potassium and calcium. The binding of acids and bases forms neutral salts. However, if our tissues are already overly acidified, one single alkaline substance will not be enough to correct the imbalance, leading to muscle and connective tissue acidification. We experience muscle soreness after athletic activities and a premature decline in performance. Excessive acidity leads to muscle and connective tissue hardening, causing tension and pain and, unfortunately, a rapidly increasing risk of injury. A good way to avoid all this is to make sure our diet supplies us with sufficient alkaline substances and to supplement it with alkaline mineral salts. Best of all is to change our nutrition so that the acid-base balance is normalized.

Acid forming foods like eggs, coffee, meat, processed meats, fish, sweets and alcohol can be equalized through an increased intake of alkaline foods like vegetables, potatoes and fruit.

Exercise in moderation boosts acid elimination, as do hot and cold showers, sauna baths, enough sleep, and lots of fresh air. Also, please try avoiding physical overstraining and emotional stress. Your meals should ideally be made up of 20 percent acid and 80 percent alkaline forming foods. Furthermore, several small meals are better than two large ones. Chew thoroughly, taking time to eat slowly and without haste. Avoid all white flower products and choose more whole food nutrition instead.

By detoxifying, we not only help our bodies to get rid of many environmental toxins, but also to eliminate chemicals harmful to our immune system and organs such as the liver, kidneys, colon, lymph glands, lungs and skin. Not only do we feel better and more alive afterwards, we also have our energy back. And we have helped our body to regain its acid-base balance. If suffering from latent or chronic acidosis, I strongly recommend a complete change in nutrition. Here Dr. K.S. proposes some further, easy and gentle detox methods:

Perfecting Your Acid-Base Balancing Act

Detoxing with Water: If you would like to do the water-detox method, drink large amounts of non-carbonated water, up to 3 liters per day, for 21 days. Your digestive tract and organs will get a complete rest and the chance to recover. All the toxins will be rinsed out of your organs.

Detoxing with Juice: During a period of 21 days, drink large amounts of freshly pressed, home-made fruit and vegetable juices. You can use cranberries, pineapple, apple, cabbage, celery, spinach and carrots. Please avoid citrus fruit, it has a higher acid content. The juice is an excellent source of nutrients and enzymes, which accelerate the detox process.

Detoxing with Herbs: Add red beets, dandelion, parsley, horsetail, gentian, goldenrod, and birch leaves to your meals. This cure will especially please your liver which will show its gratitude by functioning well again. Medical studies have shown that all these herbs are excellent contributors to detoxification. Kidneys are responsible for distributing significant amounts of toxins throughout the body. Toxins come in tangible and intangible form. For a kidney cleansing, you need dandelion and real bearberry. To detox lungs, you need black salsify and Chinese ephedra. While taking these herbs, you should absolutely avoid any fatty foods and all fast foods.

Detoxing Through Dry Skin-Brushing: Scrubbing your skin is a gentle, yet highly effective way of detoxing. It removes dead skin cells, stimulates the lymph system and removes any toxins on the skin. Use a special dry skin brush with soft bristles for this method. Also remember to brush the soles of your feet in a circular movement for one minute.

Detoxing with Saunas: Taking saunas is a very effective way to drain our bodies of any toxins that have settled in various parts of our system. For best results, I recommend it in combination with a healthy diet and lots of exercise. But, be careful! This method is not suitable for anyone with heart or circulatory problems, or any other disorders which might forbid saunas. Please be sure to consult your doctor.

Important to Know

What is actually the difference between detoxification and a cleanse? Unfortunately, the food we eat often also contains toxins, which our body stores after being absorbed by the intestines. These substances accumulate in the bones, the liver, bladder, kidneys, skin, fatty tissues and of course, in the intestines themselves, and can trigger numerous diseases. They either occur as natural waste products through the metabolic process, like acids, or are simply toxic components of our food. For example, toxic trace elements such as arsenic, lead, cadmium and mercury can be part our food, or other toxins which have been added for processing and/or storage purposes such as benzo pyrene* in smoked foods, as well as food dyes and preservatives, nitrates, pesticides, mycotoxins, packaging softeners, and tin from canned goods.

Over time, excess storage of these substances in our bodies leads to slagging and toxicity. Normally, the body's buffer system can neutralize an over-abundance of acids. If, however, this natural regulatory mechanism is no longer able to handle the excess acids, the body will resort to its available mineral substances. These are mainly potassium, calcium, magnesium and phosphorus, which, in combination with the acids, form complex salts which are stored as so-called slags, resulting in progressive body toxicity. In other words, our body is creating a kind of hazardous waste landfill in areas where proper metabolic process can no longer be achieved. This shows the importance of both cleansing and detoxifying.

---

* Benzo pyrene occurs in coal tar. Extracted from coal and other forms of tar, it is an aromatic hydrocarbon. It is also found in foods grilled over charcoal or pinecone fires, and is the result of partially burned organic materials such as wood, coals, and mineral oil and is a substance in exhaust, tobacco smoke, fried, grilled and smoked food products. Benzo pyrene is produced through heat. Testicular cancer in chimney sweeps as well as lung cancer in smokers are ascribed to benzo pyrene.

Doctor K.S.' 7-Day Detoxification Plan

When you are ready, take a week and follow this detox plan conscientiously. I'm certain the results will amaze you. And you will find how easy it is to follow the instructions.

During this time, it is absolutely vital that you drink lots of fluids, at least 4.2 pts. Please completely refrain from sparkling water, and also, until day seven, all freshly pressed fruit juices!! Start every day with a glass of non-carbonated water at room temperature! Drink water during the day, and flavor it with lemon, lime and/ or a cinnamon stick, according to your taste. You may enjoy sugar-free coffee, but without whitener, cream or condensed milk, or any kind of artificial sweetener. You can also have all black, loose leaf, and herbal teas. I recommend unsweetened matcha tea. Just remember, during this period, water is the very best thing for your body.

Should you feel hungry at any time, chia seeds will keep you satiated. You are allowed up to 4 tablespoons per day (see recipe on Day One).

Day One
1. Upon rising, start your day with 1 glass of non-carbonated water at room temperature!
2. On the menu: any and all fruit - **except bananas!**

3. During the first day, you can eat all and any fruit you like. Best of all is lots of melon, especially water melon!

On Day One, the more melon you eat, the better chance you have of losing up to 3.3 lbs.

On both Day One and Day Two, be sure to eat raw fruit. Do not cook, fry, mash or blend it. This will boost the detoxing process because the first stage of digestion begins in your mouth. Our saliva contains substances which promote digestion and activate our pancreas.

Why and How it Works
On day one, you are preparing your body for what is to come. Your only food intake is fresh fruit, which is the perfect food, offering all necessary vitamins and minerals.

Chia Seed Gel Recipe
Place a little less than 1 cup of non-carbonated water and 2 Tbsp. of chia seeds in a bowl you can seal. Please avoid plastic! Stir the contents well, so that the seeds are fully immersed. Close the top and let sit for 15 minutes. Now the chia gel is ready. If you chose to wait longer, please keep it in the fridge, sealed with the lid. Chia seeds have no taste of their own, so you can easily add them to any dish, drink, or to muesli, fruit salads, desserts, vegetables, and salads (see pages 258 and 275).

Day Two

1. Upon rising, start your day with 1 glass of non-carbonated water at room temperature!
2. On the menu: all-you-can-eat veggies
3. Today you may eat any and as many vegetables, either cooked or steamed, until you're completely full. No rules regarding the amount, but please **avoid all beans of any kind, corn, sweet potatoes, peas, chickpeas, mushrooms and pumpkin!**
4. **For breakfast**, eat one boiled potato, the size is not important. Please note that today you may have just **one** potato, not more!! For refinement, you may add some coconut oil, and/or goat or sheep butter.

Why and How it Works

Day Two starts with carbohydrates, plus a small portion of natural fat, butter, or coconut oil. In the morning, this will provide you with energy and balance. During the remainder of the day, the practically calorie-free veggies will give you plenty of nutrients and fibers.

Veggie Recipe: Wash and chop the vegetables of your choice into bite size pieces. In a wok, heat up 1 Tbsp. of coconut oil. Add some onions and garlic, then your veggies. Starting with the hardest kind first, like carrots, then broccoli etc., adding them at one minute intervals. Stir well with a wooden spoon. After another 2 minutes, add 1½ to a maximum of 3 Tbsp. oyster sauce (from your Asian market) and ½ cup of water. Stir one last time. Done, and ready to go!

Day Three

1. Upon rising, start your day with 1 glass of non-carbonated water at room temperature!
2. On the menu: all-you-can-eat fruit and veggies.
3. Today, eat a mixture of fruit and vegetables, eating as much as you can. But still **no bananas, and today no potatoes!** Again today, refrain from eating any kind of beans, corn, sweet potatoes, mushrooms and pumpkin!!

Why and How it Works

Day Three leaves off the potato, because you are getting your necessary carbohydrates from the fruit. Your body is now ready to start the process of burning off excess pounds. You may still be having certain cravings, but these should subside after today.

Day Four

1. Upon rising, start your day with 1 glass of non-carbonated water at room temperature!
2. On the menu: bananas, milk and veggie soup
3. Today, you are allowed to eat up to **8 bananas,** and drink up to 1 liter (2.11 pints or 4.1 cups) **of almond, oat, or quinoa milk.** You will combine

these meals with a special vegetable soup, which you can eat as much of as your heart desires.

You can also replace the bananas with avocado. You are allowed ½ an avocado per meal. You can also blend it with milk. **If you should opt for avocado, please eat ONLY avocado on this day! Do not eat bananas and avocados! Please choose either one or the other!**

Why and How it Works

Day Four may sound a little strange with bananas, milk and veggie soup. But you will be surprised. And will probably not even be able to eat all the bananas allowed. These are great sources of potassium and magnesium, all minerals which you have been losing in the past three days. Today you should be noticing your lack of cravings.

Veggie Soup Recipe: This soup is meant as an addition to your overall nutritional intake. After Day Four, you can eat it in unlimited doses, at any time. So please feel free to consume it in large quantities.

Wash, clean, and chop 2 green peppers, ½ head of kale, and 3 stocks of celery. Peel and cube 6 onions. Fill a large pot with approximately 4 cups of water, adding in the chopped veggies, along with 9 quartered tomatoes. Once it comes to a boil, turn the heat down to average, and let cook gently for about 20 minutes. Flavor with Himalaya salt and add fresh herbs of your choice. If you have a distaste for kale, you can replace it with fresh spinach leaves. **Careful!** Please store this soup only in the fridge and for no longer than 2 days.

Day Five

1. Upon rising, start your day with 1 glass of non-carbonated water at room temperature!
2. On the menu: beef and tomatoes
3. In the course of the day, you will have two portions of lean beef (for example 2 pieces of filet of approx. 10 oz. each) with tomatoes. You can also eat less meat, if you prefer. Each portion should be eaten along with 6 raw tomatoes. The tomatoes are the most effective when they are raw, and are neither cooked, fried nor grilled. On Day Five, you must add at least another 4 cups of water to your fluid intake! This will help eliminate the extra uric acid your body will now be producing. You may also replace the beef with chicken or fish, but please without the skin. If you dislike tomatoes, they can be replaced with lettuce instead. Of course, **vegetarians** can substitute other food (containing proteins!) for the meat. This day is important to consume proteins!!

Why and How it Works

On Day Five, your body is supplied with much needed iron and proteins, while the tomatoes help with digestion. By now, your urine should be clear and colorless.

Today's food quantity is close to the American "quarter pounder", but please do not feel under obligation to eat all this meat. On the other hand, please do absolutely eat 6 tomatoes!!!

Beef Recipe: Heat 1 Tbsp. of coconut oil in a pan and fry the meat. Season to your taste only after frying and eat with raw, sliced tomatoes. You may also boil or grill the meat.

Day Six

1. Upon rising, start your day with 1 glass of non-carbonated water at room temperature!
2. On the menu: beef and vegetables
3. Today you may eat unlimited amounts of lean beef and vegetables (but please stick to the vegetable rule, see Day Two). And you will be surprised how little this will be. You can also replace the beef with other lean meat (chicken, fish, as on Day Five), and instead of veggies, you can have salad with a simple vinaigrette.

Vegetarians can substitute other foods (containing proteins) for the meat. This day is important to consume proteins!

Why and How it Works

Day Six is pretty much the same as Day Five. The meat contains iron and protein, whereas the veggies supply vitamins and fiber. By today, your body will be showing a certain tendency to lose weight. And better yet, you will see a definite difference to the weight you started out with on Day One.

Day Seven
1. Upon rising, start your day with 1 glass of non-carbonated water at room temperature!
2. On the menu: brown rice and veggies, fruit juice
3. Today you will be eating brown rice (whole rice), freshly pressed fruit juice (Not the store-bought kind!!) and any vegetables you wish. But please do not eat white rice! If you do not like rice, you can leave it off your menu and simply eat veggies and drink various fruit juices.

Why and How it Works
Day Seven ends the program much like a Victorian meal ends with a good cigar, except in a much healthier way. You have taken good care of your body and it will certainly show gratitude for the cleansing and detoxing. This day ends the cleansing and now the fat burning process can begin. This week has helped cleanse your stomach and your entire digestive system. If you feel the need to lose some more weight, it is perfectly fine to repeat the procedure.

Vitamin Juice Recipe: Wash, clean and chop 4 small red beets, 6 middle sized carrots, and 1 apple and place into a juicer. In a glass, add several drops of cold pressed olive oil or coconut oil, pour in the juice, stir and enjoy.

Outcome: Weighing Less than a Week Ago

Today, on the morning of the eighth day, your weight will have gone done by six to eleven pounds. Provided you followed the detox plan exactly. Starting today, be sure to take your daily dose of chia seeds, either as a gel, or sprinkled dry onto your salads and veggie dishes. Or, taken shortly before a meal, they will curb your appetite: stir 2 Tbsp. of chia seed-gel into a small glass of almond or quinoa milk, and you're all set.

Important Facts

The instructions for this program are designed to enhance your eating enjoyment. Not everyone is a fan of cabbage, bell-peppers, carrots and the like. Which is why this program is flexible, allowing you to switch and replace veggies according to your taste. You can use any vegetable you like. Except, hands off all beans of any kind, they have too many calories!

- You may also eat your veggies in salad form, if you prefer. But please do not use store-bought dressings!
- Instead, for your dressing, use wine-vinegar or freshly pressed lemon juice, garlic and herbs.
- Please keep the coconut or cold pressed virgin olive oil to 1(!) Tbsp. per dressing.

- During the detox, please do not have more than two glasses of white wine per day.
- You may also substitute white wine with champagne.
- With the exception of beer, which is permitted, all other kinds of alcoholic beverages are strictly off-limits!
- All liqueurs, bourbon, vodka, rum, etc. are all forbidden!
- Creamy drinks and cocktails are especially forbidden!
- If you are in the mood for schnapps, please keep your intake to two schnapps during the entire course of the detox week.
- If you drink wine, please drink only wine on the given day. If you drink beer, then only beer. Please remember that alcohol is full of useless calories.
- Please do not discontinue the 7-day detox plan! If, for some reason, you need to interrupt it, please start over again at Day One. The specific order of the days is crucial, because without it your metabolism will not get the boost needed to initiate weight loss.
- If you feel headaches coming on during the week, and you can't seem to shake them despite enough fluid intake, you may take a pain-killer. In this case, Dr. K.S. recommends acetaminophen.

- If you should suffer from diarrhea during the detox week, which is rare, be sure to take chia gel.
- This detox plan is suitable for vegetarians and vegans alike.
- The detox plan is equally suited for people with severe illnesses. It is even recommended for cancer patients.
- If your doctor has prescribed any medication, you should continue to take it during the detox. Once it is over, I recommend seeing your physician for a check-up. He may need to reduce your medication (for example for diabetes) or adjust the dosage. This is especially important, if you are planning to change to healthy eating after the detoxification week!

Preparing for the New Way of Eating

After the first week, the detox plan will help cleanse your body, and more specifically, your digestive system and your stomach. If you wish to lose further weigh, you can repeat the process. You can repeat it as often as you like.

On Day Three and Day Four, your weight may not go down by much. Stay cool! This is pretty normal. You will be rewarded with a big A-HA by Day Six and Seven. Keep in mind that this program is designed to do two things; detox and reduce weight. The detox is to prepare your system for an effective change in diet, which will then rid you sustainably of excess weight. For this, the cleansing process is crucial. If, for example, we were to pot a plant in old, hard and dry soil, it would not flourish. No matter how much we watered it, it wouldn't work. However, if we put the plant in new, fresh and nutritious soil, it will blossom into a beautiful flower. But remember to water it! In other words, please be sure to drink plenty of water during the program. If you get a headache, or feel discomfort, or nausea, which can happen, it is a sure sign to drink more water!!!

If you wish to continue losing weight after the program, you should do the following for the next eight weeks:

- Completely avoid fast food products.
- Eat potatoes, rice and pasta mostly during the day. Not in the evening! If potatoes are on your menu, clean the skins thoroughly and eat them also, they provide fiber.
- Right after waking up, have a glass of non-carbonated water at room temperature. It's a huge boost for your elimination process.
- Avoid drinking "normal" milk.
- Eat mostly fruit and vegetables
- Have dinner before 7:00 PM. Remember, your colon goes to bed with the chickens.

This is one of the best ways to lose weight.

INCIDENTALLY: Should you feel food cravings coming on - which tend to jump on us in the evening and lead to the all-feared yo-yo effect - have a large glass of lukewarm water. You may also always have some Veggie Soup (see recipe in the 7-day detox plan on page 175). 2 to 3 Tbsp. of chia gel are permitted, or a handful of nuts (Brazil nuts or almonds), Harz cheese (also in an oil and vinegar marinade), a hard-boiled egg with Himalaya salt as well as sour pickles (best of all cornichon gherkins).

Since we have been avoiding carbohydrates in the evening, we no longer have sugar cravings. Of course, that's not always possible. For instance, when we have a dinner invitation or are simply in the mood, we will have the occasional pasta, or pizza at the Italian's around the corner, or steak, veggie and mashed potato dinner at the steak-house, or sushi at a Chinese restaurant. And with my 300-day system, this works beautifully.

The New Way of Eating According to Doctor K.S.

As I mentioned earlier in this book, there are both yea-sayers and nay-sayers on the subject of blood-type nutrition. Because I am neither a medical doctor, nor an expert in nutrition, I am not in a position to prove anything. I can, however, clearly state that this kind of diet has been wonderfully beneficial for both my husband and myself. I just wish all the arguing parties would commit to researching the subject together, for the benefit of humanity, instead of wasting precious time with vilifying and attacking each other. In World War II, Japanese soldiers were selected according to their blood types. Still today, hardly anyone is hired in Japan without the appropriate blood type, the belief being that conclusions can be drawn regarding a person's personality, character traits, and agreeability of disposition. If someone refuses to name his or her blood type, it's considered a sign of shame. It even seems customary, in private encounters, to ask the other person about their blood type, a little like we might ask a person what zodiac sign they are. It all became quite a thing in Japan. But the blood type-character-analysis did get somewhat out of hand when, in the early seventies, classrooms were put together according to the students' blood types. Today this Japanese popular belief is considered racist. *Hallelujah!*

This reminded me of the old Chinese woman's tale about finding the middle ground. But the belief in a connection between personality and blood type is not only common in Japan, but also in Korea, and in Taiwan. This may explain the 2005 success of the South Korean movie-romance called "My boyfriend is Blood Type B", in which a college girl, blood type A, suffers turbulent times with her raving and unpredictable partner.

Our Blood Speaks

Taking a closer look at the health benefits the blood type diet offers, it is easy to see why people of a certain blood type group are more susceptible to various diseases than others. It has been proven that certain pathogens tend to "attack" certain blood types. For example, in the Middles Ages, blood type A was sought out by small pox, whereas people with blood type 0 were victims of the plague. Think what you will, I personally can only emphasize, time and again, that the blood type diet according to Dr. K.S., in combination with my "300-day-system", and the regulation of our pH balance have led to fantastic results for my husband and myself.

In Germany, 41 percent of the population has blood type 0; 43 percent has blood type A; 11 percent, blood type B, and only 5 percent has blood type AB. Here in Asia, blood type B is very common, whereas in Europe, blood type A is predominant.

An American doctor by the name of James D'Adamo started research on blood types in the late fifties. He found a link between nutrition and blood types. During his studies, he noticed that some patients tolerated low fat and strictly vegetarian diets, while others did not. D'Adamo was determined to find out why. Some particularity in blood must be the cause, and offer an explanation.

For the first time, in 1972, Japanese journalist Masahiko Nomi and his son Toshitaka presented a book on the connection between character and blood type. Together, they authored 65 books on the subject.

In 1978, Bastyr University was founded in Seattle, Washington. It is the first accredited and multidisciplinary university for alternative medicine in the United States. After his mother had succumbed to breast cancer, D'Adamo's son, Peter, enrolled at this school to study naturpathic medicine. Two years later, his father published his first book on blood type nutrition. His son, Peter, wanting to make sure the work met scientific requirements, reviewed his father's findings. He soon found that his father's first studies on the link between blood types, nutrition and health were of far greater importance than he had ever imagined.

In 1989, Dr. Peter D'Adamo held the spectacular speech at the American Association of Naturpathic Physicians' annual convention in Oregon, that would cause the final breakthrough. Within a year, the major part of his father's findings on blood types was confirmed by genetic researchers. Since then the blood type diet has been implemented by numerous clinics throughout the United States. It was to take another seven years, for the concept to reach the wider American public.

Peter D'Adamo grew up in a family which predominantly had blood type A. In accordance with his father's occupation, the family's diet was mainly vegetarian, consisting of tofu, steamed vegetables, and salads. As a child, he often felt ashamed, feeling at a disadvantage because none of his friends ate "weird stuff" like tofu. They were happily settling into the new standard diet, which was conquering the United States of the fifties and consisted mainly of hamburgers, hotdogs, French fries dripping of oil, chocolate bars, ice cream, Coca-Cola and other soft drinks.

Blood type diet researchers are convinced that our blood type is the key to our entire immune system. It determines and regulates the influence which viruses, bacteria, infections, chemical substances, emotional strains and various life circumstances may have on each of us individually.

To this day, Peter D'Adamo eats the same way he did during childhood. Every day, he eats the foods specifically suited to his blood type. Of course the question remains, whether he has, as we do, the occasional "Fun Day".

A prominent newspaper's special edition on diets wrote on blood type nutrition: "Foods in contradiction with the supposedly 'natural' diet, are, according to the blood type diet, toxic. However, although we are still alive despite years of violating these rules, the question arises as to whether this diet is useful or utterly nonsensical."

My answer to this is: Nowhere is there even the slightest hint indicating that anyone should die, if they didn't comply with the blood type diet recommendations. And besides the fact that we are exposed to "real" toxins in the form of plastic, medicines, and environmental pollution on a daily basis, I find using the term "toxic" in connection with the blood type diet highly exaggerated. German consumer organization, Stiftung Warentest, pointed out on its website, yet again: German Nutrition Society (DGE) restates that there are no scientific facts backing the benefits of the so-called blood type diet." Please allow me another very personal, clarifying comment at this point. If there really were no benefits, this would obviously mean that my husband and I are merely imagining all the weight we lost, our excellent blood values, and the fact that we no longer need any medication whatsoever. Incidentally, there is a growing number of blood type nutrition followers worldwide, with thousands of testimonials. Genetic research, the German consumer organization, and the DGE merely have not yet found their common ground. Though the truth is, that the blood type diet is being used successfully in many clinics throughout the United States.

Blood Type Nutrition
According to Doctor K.S.

Although the blood type nutrition plan Dr. K.S. suggests leans heavily on Dr. D'Adamo's diet I mentioned previously, it diverges in certain ways which may end up making a significant difference.

Thanks to Doctor K.S.' stacks of reading material, along with his many lectures, we have studied the subject of blood type diets extensively and decided to stay with it - to this day.

Blood type 0 people, of which my husband is one, have different characteristics from those of the A blood type, like me. But that isn't all. There are specific foods which agree especially well with certain blood types, while being incompatible with others. Also regarding athletic activities, here the various blood types show different reactions. Mild exercising is better for some, while vigorous training is better for others.

We personally believe the blood type categorizations and characterizations to be meaningful and consistent. They support us in our efforts to sustain our good health. We also endorse Dr. K.S.' recommended diet changes along with the 300-day-system (devised by yours truly), in combination with a healthy pH balance. Eating, however, is so much more than just putting food into your body, because so many factors influence the complicated digestive process. For you to savor your meals to the fullest, I recommend following these instructions:

Digesting Your Meals with Ease

- The longer food stays in your mouth, which, by the way, also stimulates your sense of taste, and the more thoroughly you chew, the better your stomach is prepared for the digestive process. Your food will be pre-digested, so to speak.
- Drink either some time before, or after your meal, not during, otherwise the fluids will dilute your digestive juices.
- Eat slowly and with leisure, without haste or stress. According to ancient Roman wisdom, food, rest and pleasure are the secret to the art of healing.
- As is well known, excessive talking while eating makes you swallow a lot of air, which can cause unpleasant gas. So, our mother telling us "to not talk too much while eating" did have real meaning.
- You should have dinner no later than 7:00 pm, so the food does not remain in your stomach overnight. Your body is no longer able to process the calories you have ingested. Also, the intestines are no longer active after this time. Remember? The intestines go to bed with the chickens.

The only sure way to lose and maintain your weight, is to change your diet. We can confirm this through our own personal experience. Naturally, everyone should feel free to try these specific nutritional changes for themselves and form their own opinion. However, I recommend an in-depth consultation with a specialist, like a natural health practitioner, or dietician. If you are interested in a personal consultation with Dr. K.S. in Kuala Lumpur, please email me. He works with one of the world's most modern labs, which uses an especially designed method to perform extremely exact blood analyses. The analysis report even documents which organ is not functioning well, and why, and what to do about it. Needless to say, this progressive technology left us speechless.

Furthermore

"Start with the children. Give them healthy food.", Dr. K.S. declared emphatically, time and again, explaining how important it is to cook healthy food for kinder-garden and primary school children. There are many overweight Malaysian, Chinese, and Indian children here in Kuala Lumpur. His urgent appeal is not only directed at South East Asia, but at all schools worldwide. School food should consist of more fruit and vegetables, be more balanced and richer in variety. As is well known, today in Germany, every fifth child is overweight or obese, and children's diabetes is increasingly on the rise. Our grandchildren's kinder-garden and school in Berlin have spaghetti and meat balls, meatballs with ketchup, and pizza on the menu on a weekly basis. Hardly ever any vegetables. In a study by Hamburg University of Applied Sciences, half of 212 surveyed school authorities were found not meeting the quality standards recommended by the German Nutrition Society (DGE), which requires lots of whole grains, fruit and vegetables. Because it takes a certain time to deliver school meals, the quality - of vegetables especially - tends to deteriorate. Better organization on the part of schools and more parental financial involvement could help school meals be healthier and more appetizing.

His Blood Type and Mine

Now to the less spectacular nutritional advice Dr. K.S. gave regarding my husband's blood group. Blood type 0 is a meat eater. People who love meat can surely imagine how happy my significant other was when he heard the good news. For my blood type, on the other hand, meat is a no-go. Not only is blood type 0 blessed with naturally high stomach acid in the small intestine, this group also has the alkaline enzyme phosphatase, which is best designed to draw maximum nutrients from meat. Among other things, phosphatase enhances protein and fat breakdown.

Diets rich in proteins such as fish, meat, and poultry, and large varieties of fruit and vegetables agree very well with this blood type. On the other hand, type 0 should be cautious with various types of grains, legumes, and especially milk products (and cow milk in particular!) due to his rather sluggish metabolism. As for my husband's reactions, we can confirm all these facts to be true. Legumes do not really constitute a major part of his diet, and when he does eat them, they often do, in fact, cause problems. Blood type 0 people have a robust digestive tract and a resilient immune system. Their thyroid also tends to be somewhat lazy, which facilitates weight gain. Their genes, however, provide them with the possibility of being strong, slim, and productive, to enjoy a long life with an optimistic disposition. Isn't that great news? Their ancestor was a very smart, if somewhat belligerent fellow. According to the blood type theory, he is characterized as the so-called hunter. Type 0 can have a certain predisposition for inflammatory conditions causing ulcers, sores, and abscesses. Dr. K.S. told us that, as early as the 1950's, there had been findings showing twice the number of various ulcer cases in this blood type group compared to other blood types. For this blood type, a diet consisting of salt water fish, sea food, red meat, liver, kale, spinach, broccoli, chia seeds, amaranth, quinoa, cold pressed olive oil for salad dressings, and coconut oil for frying and cooking, as well as kelp would be especially beneficial. The seaweed called bladder wrack is a further excellent nutrient, and highly effective for weight control. The L-fucose it contains (not to be confused with fructose) can help normalize their slow metabolism, thereby encouraging weight loss. Besides seaweed, also supplemented vitamins B and K, calcium, iodine, and licorice all provide overall good health.

Stress has an immediate negative impact on this type's body, even causing them to react aggressively, which, in turn, directly effects their muscle tissue. The best way to diminish stress is engage in physical activity. To ensure a feeling of well-being, it is vital for this group to pursue athletic activities several times a week. It lightens their mood, raises their self-confidence and gives them balance. All this is conspicuously accurate and true of my husband. He exercises three times a week with great enthusiasm. And every time he comes home, he describes, in all manner of enticing variations, how wonderfully balanced he feels, and he urges me, time and again, to finally get with the program. And this is how Dr. K.S. explains the advantages of exercising: "The elevation of acidity in muscle tissue through exercise generates higher fat metabolism, generally known as fat burning. Suitable intense physical activities for my husband would include aerobic exercise, martial arts, running and weight lifting.

Regarding his character, he is said to be gregarious and optimistic by nature, and, thanks to his extreme bullheadedness, never to be deterred from pursuing his goals. Beneath his hard shell, lies a big heart.

Stubbornness being his middle name, this typical workaholic frowns on outside advice. Yet deep down, he is highly emotional and true to a fault, even though he has a hard time showing his feelings. According to the Japanese character trait interpretation of blood type 0, he is endowed with leadership skills, making him a natural spokesperson. He is determined, ambitious, athletic, and resilient, self-confident, and he is endowed with a large dose of logical thinking. And again, I must agree to all of the above. But one thing I do wonder about is: How is it that the Japanese know my husband so well?

I Am Type A

The problem for type A people is, as I mentioned before, meat. My stomach has a hard time digesting it, due to my lack of sufficient stomach acids. Meat makes type A sleepy and sluggish. It is hard for my body to break down fats and animal protein, because, as a member of this group, I am missing the alkaline enzyme called phosphatase. As a result, both are stored as fat reserves, metabolism is slowed down, which provokes an insulin reaction. This leads to obesity and diabetes. No contradiction from me on any of this.

On the other hand, blood type A is very good at handling fiber, Dr. K.S. explained, since my body benefits most from vegetables, fruit and corn. Further foods like chia seeds, amaranth, quinoa, cold pressed olive oil in salad dressings, and coconut oil used for frying foods work almost as effectively as curing remedies in my case.

It is said that Type A can virtually reverse the negative impact of stress, by dealing with the initial phase of it by mental, as opposed to physical, means. The down side however, that stress can accumulate in the body, causing irritability, hyperactivity, and anxiety. This can weaken the immune system to the point of opening the doors to heart disease, or even cancer, for which I already had a propensity. Anemia, type 2 diabetes, gallbladder, and liver problems; infestation of microorganisms - counting worms and parasites - are all further diseases I could be threatened by. Blood type A people can, however, counter stress with mild physical exercise such as meditation, yoga, tai-chi, swimming, hiking, and saunas. These activities provide physical relaxation, which, for this blood type, even enhances the ability to concentrate. For people of this group, more physically strenuous athletic activities - especially athletic competition - causes even more stress. As you well know, I can only agree to all of the above.

Type A people have tolerant immune systems and sensitive gastro-intestinal tracts. This is why a vegetarian diet, rich in fruit and vegetables is especially suited for me. I may eat fish several times a week. If I wish to lose weight, besides leaving off meat, I should avoid all wheat products, kidney and lima beans, and all milk products (and no cow milk, goes without saying!) Outside of very few exceptions, almost all legumes suit my blood type just fine. To be exact, I am actually more vegetarian, which is why seafood, fish, and tofu agree with me very well.

According to the characteristics of my blood type, I am said to be a shy perfectionist, true blue and compassionate, and more quiet than outgoing. I am a somewhat introverted personality, initially cautious when it comes to making acquaintances, and generally careful with anything new or unknown. These order-loving aesthetes are said to be nearly unsurpassable in all creative areas. And as sensitive perfectionists, they tend to be quite obstinate, and often find it difficult simply to relax. The reason for this is their extremely helpful nature, causing them to feel responsible for everything and everyone around them. Unfortunately, despite this being a wonderful quality, it can make this somewhat overly careful and sometimes insecure A-type personality appear pressured, tense and nervous. When they take on a task, they always give a thousand percent, which can surely be blamed on their tremendous sense of obligation. While caring about other people's opinions, this highly organized character also attaches great importance to honesty.

The Japanese character interpretation of my blood type rates me as being perfectionistic, orderly, law-abiding, obsessed with detail, industrious, idealistic, diligent, choosy, insistent, elegant, responsible and dutiful, helpful, cautious, punctual, and blessed with excellent organizational talents. You may see why I prefer not to comment on this assessment. However, there is one more thing listed. Interestingly, under "possible typical professions", the list includes writer and columnist.

The Force of Habit

"Change is a good thing, just not for me." Haven't we all heard this one before? We all make up a million excuses for NOW to be just the wrong time for a change of diet. My job! My kids! The trip we planned! After my vacation! Aunt Paula … The weather's too bad! Too hot! Too cold! Too sunny! Too stressful! But let's be honest, where there's a will, there's always a way to achieve our goals. I don't mean climbing Mount Everest, crossing the ocean in a canoe, or taking part in the next moon landing. We're only talking about simple changes. Following through on a detox week and changing our diet in a way that will allow us to lose weight successfully, stay healthy, or return to good health. Of course, most of us have strenuous jobs, families, kids - all of which can be overwhelming at times. We believe that we just don't have the time to prepare healthy breakfasts, or home-made lunches and dinners, except for maybe on weekends. But if we were truly honest, we would have to admit that this is simply not true! We could get up a little earlier, cook things in advance, and make some preliminary preparations the night before. It's all just a matter of organization. "Oh, no way! In the evening I need to relax. I've had such a hard day", was always my argument. It was much easier than changing my longstanding habits. And so convenient: just pop into the supermarket, always grabbing the same packaged, canned, and ready-made foods, without ever having to read the labels. The force of habit.

People whose serious diseases have forced them to change their way of life completely should serve as an example to us, like the person who suddenly finds him or herself in a wheel chair, on crutches, or on dialysis has been forced to change all his or her habits at once. We can be truly grateful, if we still have the choice to do so voluntarily! We chose to do it for ourselves, for our health, for feeling better in our bodies. Start eating more healthily and change your nutrition. I promise you, it's worth it! As soon as it becomes a habit, and you have conquered your weaker self, you will say: "Wow! That was easy-peasy!"

Plastic and Company

"Remove anything made of plastic from your kitchen", Dr. K.S. growled, waving a threatening index finger in front of my nose. Years ago, I had heard that you shouldn't use plastic containers to put food in the microwave. Via the food, toxic substances would be released into your system. But that isn't all. Every year, worldwide, we produce an estimated 240 million tons of plastic. It is a well-known fact today, that this non-biodegradable material causes environmental problems. However, that our kitchen utensils pose health problems and may even threaten humanity's reproduction was news to me. Of course, in this day and age, it is hardly possible to live in a completely plastic-free world. The stuff is everywhere! But regarding the kitchen, we do have some choices. We can use glass, wood, enamel, metal and ceramics.

A study found plastic residue in the blood of 95 out of 100 people tested. In an American study performed on a family of six, researchers found that damaging substances absorbed by their food from Tupperware receptacles and the like were transferred to their bodies through their meals. At the beginning of the eight-week study, all family members showed high contents of toxic substances. In the next step, all plastic objects were removed from the kitchen. The final blood analysis showed astonishing results. The toxic substances likely to cause cancer, allergies, asthma, and other serious diseases, and even testicular cancer and sperm-damage, were reduced to almost acceptable levels. The main culprits here are so-called phthalates, which, in their low molecular form (DEHP, paraben, PCB, and others) are used as softeners in plastic containers, bags, wrappers, in PVC, and numerous beverage bottles. Researchers have been sounding the alarm for some time now: DEHP - di(2-ethylhexyl) phthalate interferes with hormonal synthesis and can cause sterility or diabetes in men. These softeners occur in our daily food at concentrations far above any acceptable tolerance levels. They are contained in almost everything, even in blood transfusion bags, exhaust fumes, baby bottles, and drinking straws, and also in medicine packaging, children's toys, and in the candy coating of lozenges. These softeners can also be absorbed through our skin, from rubber boots, rain coats, body lotions, perfume, our car dash boards, diaper changing mats, and so on. I've often wondered, how is it that babies, just barely born, can already have leukemia? Could the answer be softeners? Big business is always downplaying the problem. It's time to take action and do something about it!

In our kitchen now, we have replaced almost all plastic with glass and porcelain containers and reinstated the old mason jars and enamel pots. We also avoid covering our food with saran wrap and storing it in plastic baggies. I buy much more food in glass containers and keep leftovers in them, in the fridge as well as in the freezer. After shopping, we immediately remove all the plastic wrappings, because, unfortunately, most food is still packaged in plastic.

Beware! Please take care to never leave plastic bottles in your car. Heat causes toxins to develop and be released into the fluid. These chemicals can cause cancer. Use metal or glass containers instead. And another piece of advice: please refrain from using simple wooden Chinese chop sticks. The media recently released information saying that these chop sticks are processed with toxins. A lab test showed that when submerged in liquid, within seconds, the Chinese chop sticks turned it into a yellowish, poisonous brew.

My Experience with Alternative Medicine

In 1981, I was suffering from a particularly aggressive form of rheumatism. Several of the rheumatology specialists we consulted in our despair agreed on a devastating diagnosis, and informed my parents that I had two, maybe two and a half years to live!

For someone who is supposed to have been dead for over 30 years, I feel better than ever before. It was alternative medicine, also known as complementary medicine, that helped me. The pharmaceutical chemo-bombs I was prescribed at the time would probably never have let it come to my writing this book.

Since 2004 I had an abnormal skin growth on my leg, which was no bigger than a penny, but had a tendency to get inflamed. Once I started taking papain, it vanished. But maybe also my entire change of diet, along with match tea, chia seeds, coconut oil and melatonin contributed to its disappearance. Or the combination of all these things. I would find it worthy of research for both conventional and alternative medical professionals to find out what actually made my growth disappear.

Be that as it may. From his vast alternative medical experience, Dr. K.S. has given us sometimes simple, but always effective tips for small issues and everyday aches and pains. In the following, I list a few of his tips for pain.

To Hell with the Pain
Salt for achy feet: warm foot baths with Himalaya salt are helpful.

Garlic for ear aches: drizzle 2 drops of warm garlic oil in the ear twice a day, for five days.

Cherries for joint pains and headaches: eating a bowl of cherries per day can help alleviate pain, without the stomach upset that pain killers can cause.

Peppermint for aching muscles: 10 drops of peppermint oil in a warm bath, three times a week.

Blueberries for bladder problems: take 1 cup of blueberries per day, either fresh, frozen or as juice.

Ginger for swelling, stiffness, cold, muscle and joint pains: take 1 teaspoon of chopped ginger in your meals or as tea.

Pineapple for indigestion and gas: eat some pineapple every day.

Grapes for back tension: consume grapes daily.

Tomato juice for leg cramps: drink 1¼ cup of fresh, pure tomato juice daily, for at least 10 days.

Honey quickly heals inner mouth wounds: four times a day, ingest one teaspoon of raw honey.

Cloves for tooth aches: gently chew on a clove to extract its juice. This can help keep a tooth ache and gum infection at bay for up to two hours. And then, off to the dentist you go!

Curcuma for chronic pain: add ¼ tsp. of curcuma to vegetable, poultry, rice, and meat dishes every day. Curcuma is also known as turmeric, yellow ginger, Indian saffron, and yellow root zedoary.

Horse radish for sinus infection: take 1 tsp., twice a day daily, of freshly grated horse radish, or eat as a spread on bread.

Apple vinegar for heart burn: 1 Tbsp. in a cup of water before every meal.

About Ayurveda

In one of our conversations, Dr. K.S., whose ancestry reaches back to India, told me that classical Ayurvedic medicine has traditionally been using urine treatment for over 5,000 years. Over time, entire generations of doctors gathered their medical experience to establish this field of medicine. The name Ayurveda is an ancient Indian term, composed of the two words "ayur" and "veda". "Ayur" means "life" and "veda" means "knowledge", therefore, Ayurveda means "knowledge of life". Ayurvedic medicine does not work right away, like a pain killer would, making your headache vanish ten minutes after you take it. In Ayurvedic medicine, the focus lies on the person who is ill, not on the illness. Ayurveda is a time tested, effective, and extremely complex healing system! Professor Thomas Tursz, well-known French oncologist and head of the Institut Gustave Roussy in Villejuif near Paris, was able to experience and find this to be true first-hand. He accompanied breast cancer patient Marinella (Nella) Banfis to South India, where she was fully cured. In July 2014, German TV channel ARTE aired a moving and inspirational documentary on the subject, which I would highly recommend to everyone.

The assumption is that Maharshi Charaka, known as the "father of medicine" in India, wrote down the core of traditional Ayurvedic literature, known as Charaka-Samhita, which still today, constitutes the fundamental source material. As a wandering Buddhist monk and doctor in the third century B.C., he researched the functions of digestion, of metabolism, of the immune system, and the basics of genetics. He not only described human anatomy with its various organs, but also all

360 bones, including all the teeth in the human body. Erroneously, he assumed the heart to have a hollow space. But he was correct in another aspect. The heart is the human "control center". Charaka never treated just one disease. He first undertook the study of all influencing factors, including the person's environment, before dispensing the appropriate treatment. Dr. K.S. explained it to me in very simple terms: "Westerners see their bodies as cars, that need to be brought to the shop, i.e. to the doctor, to change the spark plugs. Ayurvedic medicine takes a very different approach. Here, we need to get a complete overview before switching out any spark plugs. In other words, we look at the big picture as a whole."

The healing properties of urine, for example, are used to treat diabetes, burns, eye diseases, ear, nose, and throat disorders, skin diseases, and digestive as well as liver problems. In India, many patients considered hopeless cases are being successfully treated with self-urine therapy. In the western part of the world, urea is well known among homeopaths. All active ingredients swimming in our blood are eliminated from our bodies in the form of urine. Isn't it just a miracle, when buried mining victims are able to survive for days without water? But it doesn't necessarily take a disaster for us to make use of the "golden juice". Today, Western conventional medicine is well aware of urine therapy. Doctors are prescribing ointments containing urine. While in former times, pig urine was used for this purpose, it was later synthesized and is now contained in many urea salves. But no copy can ever reach the quality of the real thing our own body produces.

Austrian herbal expert and author Maria Treben, whose opinions are often controversial, wrote in one of her books the following inspirational statement: "Created by nature, through nature healing we shall find". The Ayurveda authors and scholars have known this for many, many centuries.

Natural Inner Beauty Tricks

Some may find this distasteful or even disgusting. Others may not. As a child, I had a wart on the back of my hand. My mother told me to put a little morning saliva on it to make it go away. So, first thing in the morning, I would run my tongue across my wart. And lo' and behold, one day it was gone. I can't recall how long it took, but, not being blessed with a lot of patience, it couldn't have been all that long.

I remembered this many years later, when I looked in the mirror and discovered the first fine lines around my eyes. Wait a minute, I thought, if my morning saliva could make my wart disappear, perhaps It could do the same with my wrinkles. So, every morning, I dabbed these little signs of age with some saliva. Later, I switched to making my own DIY anti-aging creams and masks with natural ingredients. And the great thing is, the masks are edible. In other words, they're vegan, and made without animal testing. Of course comparative advertising is forbidden, but still, many of my friends who know and use my DIY creations claim they are at least as effective as "La...", if not even a little more. But I do still spit on a Q-Tipp to remove smeared mascara.

In the mid-nineties, after reading Carmen Thomas' book "A Very Special Juice - Urine", for some time I applied morning mid-stream urine on the calluses of my feet and elbows. After just a few weeks, these areas were supple and soft. Incidentally, urine does not smell when applied to your skin, because the skin pores immediately absorb it into the body. This may sound disgusting to some people, but nevertheless, the knowledge ancient civilizations had on successful self-urine treatments was passed down through the centuries to the present. The ancient Egyptians, for instance, were masters at testing urine. Descriptions of disease diagnosis and their treatments with urine were recorded in their medical papyri. In his writings, Hippocrates also recommended using urine as a means of diagnosis as well as a therapy. In the old days, it was even common for doctors to taste a patient's urine to determine if it was sweet, which was an indication of diabetes. But do not worry, urine is sterile, except in case of kidney disease. If you are healthy, the "special juice" is germ-free. Recently, an American 15 year-old caused an uproar in cancer medicine with urine - more specifically with a test strip you had to pee on. Within minutes, the strip would show whether the person had cancer or not. In other words, our urine works like a sort of inner mirror.

BY THE WAY: More information about rejuvenation, beauty tips and recipes for self-made tonics, masks, creams, lipsticks etc. you'll find in my new book "SOS - Schön ohne Schummeln", published in 2017 by Goldmann / Random House, ISBN: 978-3-442-22180-6 WG 2463.

How We're Doing Today

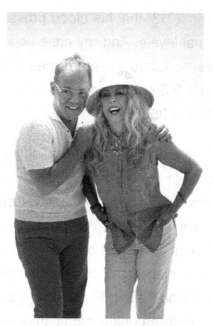

Katharina and Husband Norbert: "Together
we are 121 years old!" (2017)

Just like in the movies, our story has a happy ending - while hopefully, of course, the end of our lives is still far, far away. And, considering the state of our health today, our chances are looking pretty good.

Back in the summer of 2010, my husband's blood pressure was more than alarming. One morning, he was feeling really terrible and went to our family doctor in Dubai. His blood pressure was 190 to 110 (systolic/diastolic pressure). Before letting him leave, the doctor immediately gave him nitrospray. The medication he prescribed after that, (co-diovan 160mg/12,5mg) failed to produce satisfactory results. His blood pressure would simply not go below 150 to 100. It was not before we saw Dr. K.S. in 2013, that his blood pressure gradually reached normal levels. And my case was no different. In Dubai, despite blood pressure medication (Exforge HCT 5/160mg/12,5mg) I was consistently stuck at an average of 140 to 95.

When our family doctor in Dubai diagnosed my high blood pressure in the spring of 2010, he said to me: "Time is running out, dear Katharina. You are on the verge of becoming diabetic. We must act immediately!" Whenever I went for a pedicure, I was always asked whether I was a diabetic, because often the procedure was a pretty bloody affair. But I always said no; I had no idea of the threatening signs that my body was obviously manifesting. I was never especially thirsty.

On the contrary, my fluid intake was actually too low. Nor were any of the other common symptoms of developing diabetes apparent. I had only this awful business with my feet, which I attributed to overly thin skin in that area. This turned out to be a huge mistake. At that time, my fasting blood sugar on awakening was 164 milligrams per deciliter (mg/dl), or 9.1 mmol/L. At first, the new medication did not agree with me. It took almost five months for the dosage to be properly adjusted. And even then, my blood sugar was never at an optimal level. I seemed stuck at an average 135 to 140 mg/dl (7.8 mmol/L).

Today, I eat practically just as much sweet food as I did before my diabetes illness, and I promise you, I had quite the sweet tooth. Changing my diet has opened countless doors to new, natural and tasty alternatives. However, despite everything, I would like to emphasize that the less sweets you indulge in, the better it is for your health!

Our Lab Results in Comparison

Blood Pressure

Optimal blood pressure: 120 / 80

Grade 3 Hypertension: 180 / 110 and more

Dangerously high blood pressure can cause stroke as well as lead to cardio-vascular disease and even death.

My current blood pressure average: 116 / 74

My husband's current blood pressure average: 125 / 85

Neither of us on medication!

Cholesterol Levels

LDL Cholesterol: < 2.58 mmol/L (< 100mg/dl)*

HDL Cholesterol: > 1.03 mmol/L (> 40 mg/dl). The sum of these values equals the total cholesterol value, should be < 5.20 mmol/L (< 202 mg/dl).

My total cholesterol level:

Before: 6.12 mmol/L (238mg/dl)

Today: 4.28 mmol/L (166 mg/dl)

My husband's total cholesterol level:

Before: 6.48 mmol/L (525 mg/dl)

Today: 3.64 mmol/L (141mg/dl)

LDL Cholesterol Levels

Ideal: < 2.58 mmol/L (< 100 mg/dl)*

Borderline: 3.3 to 4.1 mmol/L (128 to 159 mg/dl)

Very high: over 4.9 mmol/L (> 190 mg/dl)

My LDL Cholesterol level:
Before: 4.14 mmol/L (161 mg/dl)
Today: 2.65 mmol/L (103 mg/dl)

My husband's LDL Cholesterol level:
Before: Unable to calculate as triglycerides are higher than 4.5 mmol/L!
Today: 1.69 mmol/L (65 mg/dl)

<u>**HDL Cholesterol Levels**</u>
Ideal: > 1.03 mmol/L (> 40 mg/dl)*
Bad for men: < 1 mmol/L (< 40 mg/dl)
Bad for women: < 1.28 mmol/L (< 50 mg/dl)

My HDL Cholesterol level:
Before: 1.02 mmol/L (39 mg/dl)
Today: 1.45 mmol/L (56 mg/dl)

My husband's HDL Cholesterol level:
Before: 1.06 mmol/L (41 mg/dl)
Today: 1.24 mmol/L (48 mg/dl)

<u>**Triglyceride Levels**</u>
Ideal: < 1.7 mmol/L (< 150 mg/dl)*
Very elevated: > 5.6 mmol/L (> 500 mg/dl)

My triglyceride level:
Before: 1.98 mmol/L (175 mg/dl)
Today: 1.45 mmol/L (128 mg/dl)

My husband's triglyceride level:
Before: over 4.52 mmol/L (> 400 mg/dl)
Today: 1.56 mmol/L (138 mg/dl)

Blood Sugar

Normal fasting blood sugar level: 3.3 to 5.5 mmol/L (60 to 100 mg/dl*)
Non-diabetic level: below 6.1 mmol/L (below 110 mg/dl)
Borderline: 5.5 to 6.6 mmol/L (100 to 120 mg mg/dl)
Diabetic: over 6.7 mmol/L (120 mg/dl) after multiple readings

My fasting blood sugar:
Before: 9.1 mmol/L (164 mg/dl)
Today: 4.7 to 4.9 mmol/L (86 to 90 mg/dl) without medication!

Note: Dr. K.S. hammered this one rule into our heads: "A high HDL cholesterol level is an advantage, and a low LDL cholesterol level sounds promising".

All values quoted are based on the blood analysis reference range provided by Dr. K.S. The values referred to as "before" were mostly samples from approximately ten months prior to the "today" values. The today values are from June 2014.

---

* mg/dl (milligram per deciliter), mml/L (millimol per liter) < (lower than), > (higher than)

Doctor K.S.: "Just Do It!"

Doctor K.S. is a perfectionist. Born in Malaysia, as the oldest of four children, he grew up in a family with the means to enable all siblings to attend medical school. The young Sikh showed a certain disposition for athletics as a child. However, he always had to be the very best at whatever he undertook. "Unfortunately, I was never really successful in sports." He had a passion for soccer, hockey and taekwondo. "But I never excelled in any of these sports." Then, later, he wanted to become a pilot. Once at university, his interests shifted again. Now he was looking into studying "something along the lines of economics". But his parents had other plans for him. He was to become a doctor, the same as all his siblings. He did not like this one bit. "My father even had to bribe me to sign up for medical school." The day finally came shortly before his 19th birthday and he enrolled at the Kasturba Medical College in Mangalore, in India. Namesake of this famous medical school was Kasturba Gandhi, wife of Mahatma Gandhi.

Just five years later, he passed his exams and practiced medicine for a year in the prominent harbor city of Mangalore, located in the southern Indian state of Karnataka, before returning home to Malaysia. From this time on, he started loving his profession. His path led him to the well-known General Hospital in Kuala

Lumpur, and later, to the General Hospital of Kuantan in northern Malaysia, where he worked in the orthopedic department. Here he was offered a residency and the chance to specialize in emergency medicine. "It was the work in emergencies that made me fully understand what it means to be a doctor."

When Doctor K.S. was given the opportunity to lead a medical team in Ulan Bator in Mongolia, he immediately interrupted his residency and accepted. His assignment there turned out to be one of his greatest challenges. "It was simply impossible to provide the best care for these patients. Practically everything was lacking." Doctor K.S. had failed in his ambition to perform at his very best. Deeply disappointed, he returned to Malaysia. There he faced difficulties reentering his residency for specialty training, which prompted him to look for a private practice. His search was successful, and soon he partnered in a shared practice with a former fellow university student. In 2004 he was able to take over the practice. "We had very different views on how medicine should be practiced today. I wanted nothing less than the best care for my patients." Shortly after, his father, who had been having heart problems for some time, was brought to the National Heart Institute, one of Malaysia's best cardiology clinics, perhaps even the best in all of Southeast Asia. Just days later, he suffered a stroke. "I was, of course, very upset that a stroke was possible in such a first rate hospital, and that despite constant observation, treatment, and good doctors. At that moment I knew something was missing in the method of treatment. I began to grasp that what I had learned at university could not be enough. Consequently, I committed to intense studies on nutritional science, alternative healing methods, and geriatrics. I found out that revitalizing medicine as well as nutritional science were the key to many, if not almost all diseases. With a special detoxification plan, customized dietary changes, targeted supplements and hormones, I was able to bring my father back to full health. With this method, and to this day, I treat all my patients, who listen carefully and follow my recommendations. I dedicate all my time to expanding my knowledge on the effects various foods have on our bodies to help my patients regenerate and gain excellent health. However, only those able to listen to their bodies and willing to change their eating habits and life-styles in a manner that goes above and beyond are sure to succeed. Eating fresh, home-cooked meals is the only right and healthy way to lose weight! Many people think it impossible to prepare home-made meals on a daily basis, or feel they simply don't have the time. But I can assure you, that once you are accustomed to it, you will realize very quickly that your body is not only losing weight, but has much more energy. But the most important change you will notice, is an overall sense of physical and emotional well-being, thanks to your healthier life-style. Your body will be grateful. It really isn't that hard. Just do it!"

Yours truly,

Doctor K.S. (July 2014)

Last, But Not Least ... by Norbert Bau

To begin with, I would like to encourage you to read this chapter with as much interest as the previous ones. And my valid argument supporting this suggestion is that I am the person in this book repeatedly referred to as "my husband" - the very same who has been faithfully following the writing, while eating, and drinking, and experiencing much of what was described in these pages. Perhaps some of you were beginning to wonder whether this "husband" even existed. But I can assure you, yes, I really do exist. To be exact, for 26 years now, I have been the so-called better half of this vivacious woman.

To cut to the chase, since my first encounter with Dr. K.S., thanks to my new healthy diet, I have slimmed down from 234 lbs to 180.7 lbs, and am enjoying an utterly new quality of life. Before meeting him, my metabolic age was that of an 80 year-old man, in other words 20 years older than I was at the time. After all his treatments and my consistent implementation of his instructions, my metabolic age has jumped back to age 51. In other words, he rejuvenated me by a whopping 29 years. Aren't mathematics just wonderful?

In the photos on left, you see one and the same person, namely me, before and after. I struggled for a long time with whether or not to give my wife permission to publish this atrocity (I mean the left one). Actually, it was our daughter who picked out this nasty snapshot (she should be disinherited for that). Be that as it may. Since the other picture portrays me as a more youthful and vibrant person, I finally caved and consented to my being outed. Let the world know how supersized I once was. But seriously; had anyone told me a year ago that someday I would be racking my brain about which foods were good or bad for me, and why, or, how, and with which ingredients to prepare our meals to provide our bodies with the necessary substances to lose our excess fat and to function properly, I would have simply called him crazy. I am not easily convinced. Just ask my wife! Maybe this all sounds terribly complicated to you, but it really isn't.

It all started when I changed doctors, due to our move from Dubai to Kuala Lumpur. My weight and my measurements didn't really bother me all that much. As the German saying goes "one grows with the task". And I had obviously seized every opportunity for growth. I had long since banned the terrible word "obesity" from my vocabulary, preferring to believe that "what you don't know, won't hurt you." Ultimately, it's not all that difficult to dress, stand, sit, or have your picture taken and look halfway decent. Besides, pants and shirts come in all sorts of sizes. You shouldn't always wear the same clothes forever anyway. I had also long since come to terms with all the pills I was taking to balance my blood pressure and cholesterol levels, to regularly lower my uric acid levels to improve my liver values, and fight my allergies. Our family doctor in Dubai, an extremely friendly, dedicated, and conscientious medical professional had already diagnosed the beginnings of fatty liver disorder and was constantly warning me to lose weight, to generally eat less meat, salt my food sparingly, basically stay away from alcohol, and take up regular exercise. And, that if I followed all these rules, I would gradually be able to improve my health. The only disorder we could not cure, was my hypertension because this was due to a genetic defect, which, however, according to him, could easily be adjusted with medication. Initially, I was not exactly thrilled by the prospect of having to take medication for the rest of my life. But my doctor reassured me that, first of all, millions of people were in the same situation and that even he himself was affected although he was much younger than I was. Well, he is a doctor after all, I persuaded myself, he must know. By a hair, I managed to balance my blood pressure to a barely tolerable level and conveniently ignored everything else. I actually didn't really feel that bad. But to ease my conscience, I bought tons of supplements - of course, only at the pharmacy. This was my strategic plan of attack.

But then, as mentioned before, came our move from Dubai to Kuala Lumpur. Our moving company did all the seaworthy packing. However, tying up the remaining countless loose ends was enough to make me wish for a big "poof!", that would just magically set up all our belongings in their proper place in Kuala Lumpur. We have moved many times in our lives - I think to more than 15 news homes. But this time, I deeply wanted it to be our last move. After all, I wasn't getting any younger. This is what I believed at the time, and it consoled me regarding my deteriorating vitality.

When the 40-foot container was sealed in front of our house, I already dreaded the day it would arrive in Kuala Lumpur. Dear God, I just wish it were all over. For the first time in my life, I felt utterly exhausted. And that's what bothered me the most. The container arrived, and just a few months later I stumbled into Dr. K.S.' office. As so often in the last ten years, I was debilitated by a bad case of flu ... and from here on, you know the rest of the story as my wife told it. What fascinated me about Dr. K.S. was that he ultimately changed me back into a fully healthy person, with flawless blood values, with quite an athletic figure, and an (almost) ideal body weight. What personally interested me the most about his diagnostics, was the fact that he saw all health problems as a consequence of a deficient diet. This means that for decades my body was not being provided with enough of the nutritional substances (minerals, vitamins, enzymes etc.) it needed to keep all the organs functioning optimally. Simply put, this led to an increasingly malfunctioning metabolism, which in turn, as mentioned before, caused elevated blood pressure, cholesterol imbalance, and high uric acid levels, low energy, poor sleep, snoring, allergies, hormonal imbalance, digestive problems and obesity. I was also astonished when Dr. K.S. told me, that even without my telling him anything about my condition, he had already seen the up-coming catastrophe in my blood analysis, and that he was further able to see my physical future - how things would have ended for me. Definitely not well. And his most important statement was that he would be able to reverse and eliminate all the damage, and this without conventional medication, but instead with specific, targeted measures. One of the "damages" he intended to eliminate was my high blood pressure which my Dubai doctor had ominously diagnosed as a genetic defect.

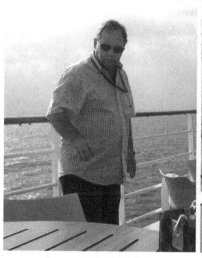 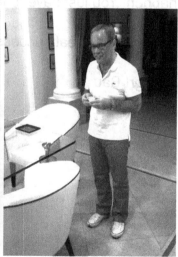

2013 – 108 Kilo   2014 – 82 Kilo

And Dr. K.S. was right in the end! For this I am very grateful. Especially for inspiring me to completely turn my eating habits and life-style up-side down. For me personally, the detox week, the dietary changes, and supplements constitute part one, while healthy foods and ingredients for cooking and baking, along with targeted exercise (as opposed to my wife) constitute part two of the plan. In my view, the combination of both parts is necessary, because it is this two-prong approach that guarantees maintaining your new sustainable sense of wellbeing. And who would of thought that one day my baggy, old, over-seized T-shirts would no longer be fit to be worn at the gym. That wasn't going to happen ...

To all my skeptical friends, I can only say: YES! It can happen! You just have to let it.

Wishing you great success,

Norbert Bau

KATHARINA BACHMAN EDITION

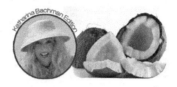

First-Rate Products For Your Transformation!

Many foods and supplements have been introduced and
described in the book, that you've just read.
Those are important, so as to carry out a successful detox week,
followed by dietary changes and adjustments to your eating habits.

Vitalingo's Katharina Bachman Edition offers a selection of those
products, which are now online available in 26 countries.

For further details you may visit our website:
https://www.sos-exercise-schmexercise.com/products

Your transformation
may begin ...

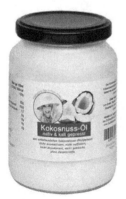

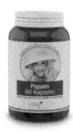

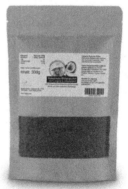

Coconut Oil   Papain Capsules   Coconut Blossom Sugar:
The Original From The Tropics

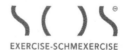

PART II

Homemade from Scratch

Katharina's Coconut Deodorant

Yields approx. 50 g (1.8oz.)

1 tsp. pure natron (sodium carbonate)

1 - 2 Tbsp. distilled water

3 Tbsp. body lotion (of your choice)

1 Tbsp. coconut oil

1 tsp. cooking starch

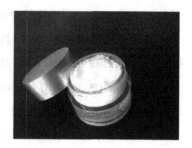

1. In a small bowl, dissolve natron (sodium carbonate) in distilled water. Add body lotion, stirring until well blended.
2. Next, add coconut oil, stir some more until mass is smooth.
3. Move mixture into small pot, sift starch through sieve and add to mass. With a metal whisk, stir constantly and heat up briefly.
4. Quickly remove from heat and continue to whisk. As soon as a firm, pudding-like consistency is reached, set aside to cool. Fill ready coconut deodorant mass into a small jar and seal. Also makes a very nice present.

Tip: Adding a little more distilled water will make the mixture more liquid, so you can fill it into roll-on deodorant bottles.

Bath Oil

Pour coconut oil into small silicon moulds and refrigerate to harden. Or, also add bits of Himalaya salt into mould before adding the oil.

Dipping an orchid or any other blossom of your choice in coconut oil and refrigerating it is also very nice and can be added to your bath.

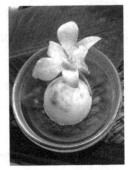

Info: Coconut oil begins to harden and turn white at temperatures below 25 degrees (77 degrees Fahrenheit). This has no influence on its quality. To liquefy the oil, simply place the sealed container in hot water.

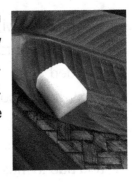

Vegetable Soup
Yields 4 Servings
2 green bell peppers
9 fresh tomatoes
½ mid-sized head of kale
3 celery sticks
6 large onions
1 bunch of fresh herbs of your choice
Spices, pink Himalaya salt

1. Wash and chop peppers, tomatoes, kale and celery. Cut tomatoes in quarters. Peel and dice onions.
2. Fill large pot with 1 l (4.2 cups) of water, add chopped veggies and bring to a boil. Turn heat down to medium and let cook gently for 20 minutes.
3. Rinse and shake herbs dry. Remove leaves from stems, chop finely and add to soup. Flavour with salt. When refrigerated, this soup will keep for 2 days.

Tip: If you prefer, instead of kale, fresh spinach leaves taste just as good in the soup. Before adding, rinse spinach thoroughly and let drip dry.

Baking Powder
Yields approx. 180 g (6 oz.)
24 g (0.85 oz.) cooking starch
65 g (2.3 oz.) (crystalline) citric acid
15 g (0.52 oz.) silicon (silica or siliceous earth)
75 g (2.64 oz.) sodium carbonate (or pure natron)

Blend all ingredients well and store, sealed in a glass or porcelain container in a dry place. Sometimes, it can clump. If it does, simply sift through sieve before use.

Tip: Please be sure never to replace citric acid with ascorbic acid. When heated to high temperatures, it breaks down into threonic acid and can cause vitamin C deficiency. A very good alternative to baking powder is tartaric acid. It's healthier, easier to digest, phosphate-free, and obtainable in almost any pharmacy.

Other ways to make baking powder

With vinegar and sodium carbonate
In the old days, bakeries made their own baking powder out of vinegar and sodium carbonate:
In a ladle, mix 1 tsp. white vinegar at 6% with 2 - 3 Tbsp. (depending on ladle size) sodium carbonate (pharmacy bought) and stir. Wait for mixture to foam and as soon as the bubbles subside, your baking powder is ready.

With sodium carbonate and tartaric acid
Blend 1 tsp. baking powder, ¼ tsp. natron and ½ tsp. tartaric acid. Because while mixing, the ingredients tend to react to one another quickly, work swiftly into your dough and bake, so as not to lose rising effect.

With sodium carbonate and acid
For 1 tsp. baking powder, mix ¼ tsp. natron with 1½ tsp. of vinegar or lemon juice.

Coconut Oil
Good quality coconut oil is obtainable in organic health food stores and Asian markets, or on the internet. You can also - by either hot or cold process - make your own homemade oil from scratch. The important thing is to use ripe, brown coconuts because these contain the most oil.

Coconut oil is very rich in antioxidants, which is why it has a long shelf life, without turning rancid. It is best to keep it in a cupboard at room temperature. Stored in the fridge, it hardens and turns white, which does not affect its quality.

In the following, I will use three coconuts in each of the two recipes, to obtain approximately 50 - 60 ml (1.69 - 2.02 fl. oz.) of coconut oil.

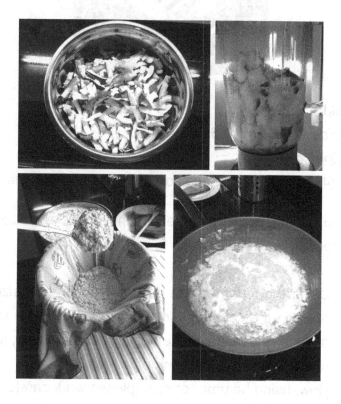

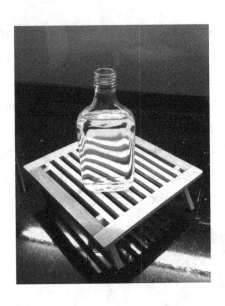

Cold & Smooth (cold pressed process)
Yields 50 - 60 ml (1.69 - 2.02 fl. oz.)
3 ripe coconuts
1 l (4.2 cups) non-carbonated water (at room temperature)

Also hammer or saw, nail, blender and clean cheesecloth, or loosely woven linen dish towel.

1. Using the hammer and nail, make two good sized holes in the coconut shell. Drain coconut juice into a glass or porcelain receptacle. (Save as drink, it is not used in the oil-making process.)
2. Now, using hammer or saw (please work carefully!) crack coconut shell open and into pieces, then remove coconut meat from inside with a strong metal spoon. Cut larger parts into smaller pieces.

3. Along with half your non-carbonated water, place coconut meat into a strong blender, making sure it is only half full. Chop first at medium, then blend at full speed to purée.
4. After covering an adequately large glass or porcelain bowl with a clean cheesecloth, place portions of coconut puree on it in steps. Once all the puree is gathered, place full cloth over a second bowl and press out liquid, which is now the coconut milk, and save in a separate jar and seal. To obtain more milk, add a little new water to the purée and repeat the blending process.
5. Store jar with coconut milk in a warm place for 12 hours, or wrap in a blanket. The jar may not be moved for 12 hours. After 12 hours, three layers will have formed: top layer is a white pulpy mass, the middle is a thin layer of oil, and at the bottom of the jar is a large quantity of milky liquid.
6. Carefully open lid and gently remove white top layer mass with a spoon and save to use otherwise (see tip). Using a second spoon or small ladle, very carefully ladle out the oil layer into a bowl. Strain oil several times, either through a very fine metal sieve or the cheesecloth (it will drip through slowly), filtering it until crystal clear. Save to a sealable glass container.

Hot and Patient (heated process)

1. As in cold pressed method, extract coconut nut meat from its shell. Heat 1 l (4.2 cups) non-carbonated water to approx. 80 degrees (176 degrees Fahrenheit). Take half of heated water and half of coconut meat and blend. As described above, squeeze milk out of pureed meat mass.

2. Next, pour coconut milk in a non-stick pan and bring to a boil. Lower to medium and let simmer until small, hard, brown coconut residue forms in the pan, from the surface of which the oil has separated. This process can take over an hour. Please do not stir during this time! With a wooden spoon, push any residue from the edges back into the bubbling mass in the middle of the pan.

3. Once reduced, strain the oily liquid through a fine metal sieve. Next, pour the oil several times through the cheese cloth (it will drip through slowly), filtering it until it becomes crystal clear. For storing, pour into sealable glass jars or bottles.

Tips

- Save the hard, brown coconut residue, you can use it to make a delicious sweet coconut sandwich spread. Simply add a roll of gula-malacca (or 150 g /5.3 oz. of coconut blossom sugar) to the pan and, while letting simmer, stir constantly until creamy. Put into mixer for final thorough blending. Fill into glass jars, and let cool. Only then, seal with tops. Refrigerated, this spread keeps for months.

- To make coconut flakes or flour, you can use the mass remaining in the cheesecloth. The longer you blend the water-coconut mixture, the finer it becomes. Spread the pressed mass onto a baking pan and dry in the oven at about 80 degrees (176 degrees Fahrenheit) for 2 to 3 hours, or longer, if necessary.
- Baking with coconut oil makes your cakes, cookies and pie crusts wonderfully light, with a delicate aroma.

Coconut Milk
Yields up to 400 ml (1.69 cups), depending on whether you repeat the process or not.

1 ripe brown coconut
Also blender, hammer or saw, nail, clean cheesecloth, or loosely woven linen dish towel.

1. Using the hammer and nail, make two good sized holes in the coconut shell. Drain coconut juice into a glass or porcelain receptacle.
2. Now, using hammer or saw (please work carefully!) crack coconut shell open and into pieces, then

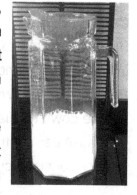

remove coconut meat from inside with a strong metal spoon. Cut larger parts into smaller pieces.

3. Place coconut flesh and coconut water in mixer and blend thoroughly at highest speed for 4 minutes. If necessary, add 100 - 150 ml (3.3 - 5 fl. oz.) non-carbonated water and continue.

4. Spread cheesecloth over adequately seized glass or porcelain bowl and spoon coconut purée onto cloth. Squeeze liquid out of purée mass into second bowl. To make more milk, please repeat the process, while adding some more water.

Tip: Coconut milk is best when used right away. However, when refrigerated in a sealed, airtight glass or porcelain receptacle, it will keep for up to 2 days. If it hardens due to cooling, just stir in some non-carbonated water or coconut water to liquefy.

Coconut Cream
Place coconut meat and water in blender and blend until creamy. Strain through metal sieve, and presto! Done!

Coconut Butter
Place 400 g (14 oz.) unsweetened organic coconut flakes in mixer and blend at highest speed for 20 minutes. Periodically, you will need to turn off your blender and scrape down the flakes stuck on the blender bowl sides with a rubber spatula. As soon as the mass reaches a buttery consistency, fill into jars and refrigerate.

Tip: Before blending, add 2 - 3 Tbsp. coconut flower sugar to the flakes. You will obtain a delicious, sweet filling for cakes, cookies and other delicacies. Sweet coconut butter tastes great as a sandwich spread or, when melted in a water bath, as a hot sauce on your favourite ice cream.

Almond Milk (Almond Milk, Unflavoured)
Yields approx. 600 - 700 ml (20 - 23.6 fl. oz.)
200 - 220 g (7 - 7.7 oz.) raw, untreated almonds

1. Rinse almonds in a bowl with fresh water, changing the water several times, thoroughly rubbing the almonds in your hands.
2. Soak almonds in filtered water for 8 -12 hours, then drain and peel off almond skins. Put in blender, adding 700 ml (20 fl. oz.) of filtered water and blend well.
3. Slowly pour mass through a metal hair sieve and strain into a bowl. Press remaining milk through sieve, or place mass in cheesecloth and squeeze out remaining milk.

Fill almond milk into glass or glass bottle and store in refrigerator for 4 - 7 days. Shake or stir well before serving.

Tip: To peel almonds easily, douse with hot water (not too hot!) and rub skin off between your fingers.

To sweeten, add coconut flower sugar, agave syrup or pitted dates to the almonds when blending.

Vanilla Flavored Almond Milk
According to taste, add vanilla extract or vanilla powder, before blending almonds.

Cinnamon Flavored Almond Milk
Add ½ tsp. cinnamon powder into mixer before blending.

Coconut Almond Milk
Thoroughly rinse 250 g (8.8 oz.) almonds and soak for 8 - 12 hours 1 l (4.2 cups) of filtered water. Drain and skin almonds. Place peeled almonds and coconut water of 3 fresh coconuts into blender. If you like, you can add 2 - 4 pitted dates or 1 Tbsp. coconut flower sugar. Blend thoroughly.

Slowly pour mass into metal hair sieve and let drip into a bowl, pressing out remaining liquid from the sieve in the end. Or, place mass into cheesecloth and squeeze out remaining milk. Fill coconut almond milk into glasses or glass bottle and consume within the day. Stir or shake well before serving.

Tip
- Instead of filtered water, you can also mix the almond milk with the water the almonds soaked in.
- Peeling the almonds is not necessarily a must.
- For lesser quantities of almond milk, use 2 Tbsp. almonds to ½ l (2.1 cups) of water.

- The left-over, squeezed out almond pulp (with or without skin) is great for baking cookies and cakes and also tastes good in muesli.

Pandan Essence

Rinse 15 - 20 dark green pandan leaves well (find at Asian market or on internet) and cut off light tips. Using scissors, cut 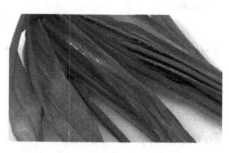 into little pieces. Place into blender with 150 ml (5 fl. oz.) water and blend at highest speed for 3 - 4 minutes, adding water if necessary. Strain green liquid, fill in airtight glass, and refrigerate for 2 days. Next, with a medical syringe or pipette, remove lighter green top layer in glass, it is bitter. Refrigerated, pandan essence keeps for 2 - 4 weeks. Throw out when it develops a strong smell.

Maybe Butter

Mix coconut oil with various foods of your choice and place in the fridge. For example ...

Tomato Butter

Stir 1 Tbsp. of tomato concentrate (per 100 g /3.5 oz.) in coconut oil and sprinkle it with taste-enhancing Himalayan salt or herbs for refinement.

Mushroom Butter

Kneed in 1 - 2 Tbsp. of sautéed mushrooms (per 100 g / 3.5 oz.). Refine with Himalayan salt and herbs of your choice.

You can also use all kind of goat or sheep butter to add foods of your choice!

Honey Substitute
To make approx. 50 - 60 ml (1.7 - 2 oz.)
300 ml (10.3 oz.) non-carbonated water
12 pandan leaves (obtainable at Asian markets or on internet)
1 roll gula-malacca (or 200 g / 7 oz.) coconut blossom sugar, or brown sugar)

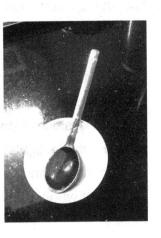

1. Fill saucepan with water and tie knots in pandan leaves. Place 6 of the pandan leaves, with gula-malacca into water and bring to a boil, occasionally pressing leaves with a wooden spoon.
2. After 15 minutes, remove leaves from water and place remaining 6 pandan leaves in saucepan for 15 minutes. The leaves should not be boiled longer than 15 minutes, otherwise they turn bitter.

3. After removing leaves, reduce liquid to syrup. This can take up to 45 minutes. Stir occasionally. Let syrup cool for 5 minutes before pouring into sealable jar. This honey substitute crystallizes after a few days, but this has no negative impact on quality.

Tip: Instead of pandan leaves, you can also use pandan essence (please see page 241) to add to the sugar. The honey substitute is also delicious when pepped-up with some organic lemon or orange zest, or other flavoring agents such as pine or fir needle, vanilla, cinnamon and many more essences.

Chocolate
Yields approx. 15 candy cups, depending on size
90 ml (3 oz.) cocoa butter
60 g (2 oz.) organic cocoa powder (70% cocoa content)
60 g (2 oz.) organic honey
1 - 1½ Tbsp. real vanilla extract
nuts of your choosing, orange or mint essence
chili powder, if desired

1. Place cocoa butter in a bowl, and melt in a water bath while stirring. Please be careful not to let any of the water get into the cocoa butter.
2. Once fully melted, remove bowl from water bath. Add cocoa powder, honey and vanilla extract to cocoa butter and stir until smooth.

3. You can flavor liquid chocolate to your heart's content, for example with roasted, finely chopped nuts of any kind, orange or mint essence, or chili powder. Spoon chocolate mass into candy cups or on baking tray lined with baking parchment.
4. Let chocolate set and harden at room temperature for 2 hours. Then refrigerate. Remove from candy cups before serving or cut to size, place in boxes or package otherwise. Chocolate keeps for over a week at room temperature, and much longer when refrigerated.

Tip: You may also switch the fat with oil, for example, or instead of honey, for example, use sugar. Just be sure to keep the ratio 90ml/60g/60g (3 oz./2 oz./2 oz.) in mind, in other words, 90 ml (3 oz.) coconut oil, 60 g (2 oz.) cocoa powder and 60 g (2 oz.) sweetener. Because it doesn't dissolve in water, the coconut flower sugar, for example, needs to be reduced to syrup beforehand, by mixing 60 g (2 oz.) sugar with 5 Tbsp. of water, bringing this to a boil and letting simmer for 10-15 minutes. Set aside to cool, then add and stir into oil-cocoa powder mixture.

My Best Recipes

Helpful Recipe Tips
Here is some useful information to begin with, which I hope you will read carefully!

- In the following recipes, you can replace almond milk, coconut, quinoa, rice or oat milk, as well as coconut blossom sugar, coconut blossom Nectar, natural agave syrup (please pay attention to the highest quality), Manuka honey, pitted dates; crystal, rock and Himalaya salt, as well as vegan cream, if need be, with "normal" ingredients.
- When using natural salts, please be aware that they are much stronger than standard table salt.
- To have good quality water for use in the following recipes I recommend filtered or non-carbonated water in glass bottles. Please refrain from buying water in plastic bottles!
- For fried dishes, whether veggies or meat, 1 Tbsp. of coconut oil is usually sufficient. Please do not use margarine!
- In certain recipes for sweets, you may replace coconut oil with butter (also homemade butter from page 241).
- All measurements in the recipes are meant as guidelines.
  - Tbsp. = tablespoon
  - tsp. = teaspoon
  - 1 cup = 180 ml (6 fl. oz.)
  - 3 Tbsp. water = 50 ml (1.7 fl. oz.)
  - 1 Tbsp. chia seeds = 12 g (0.4 oz.)
  - 100 ml (3.4 fl. oz.) water and 12 g (0.4 oz.) chia seeds = 1 egg

Making Chia Seed Gel

In some of the following recipes, I use chia gel, which is gelled chia seeds. In a glass or porcelain receptacle, stir 1 Tbsp. chia seeds into 100 ml (3.4 fl. oz.) non-carbonated water and let swell for 15 minutes, or longer, which makes their nutritional ingredients even easier to metabolize. Refrigerated, the gel can keep for up to 5 days. Stir before using. If you consume dry chia seeds, please make sure your water intake is sufficient, because the little seeds absorb a lot of fluid. The US Health Department recommends eating no more than 48 g (1.7 oz.) of dry seeds per day.

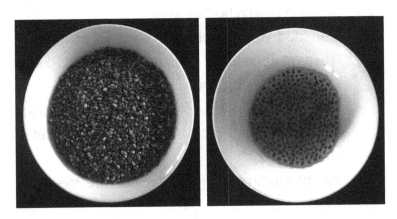

Chia Egg Substitute

To replace one egg: Let 1 Tbsp. chia seeds swell in 100 ml (3.4 fl. oz.) non-carbonated water for 15 minutes. Next, put in blender and blend well, until a white, pudding-like mass has formed. Add water by the spoon, if needed.

How to Cook Amaranth

Cook amaranth at a ratio of 1 to 2. In other words, let 200g (7 oz.) amaranth come to a boil in 400 ml (14 fl. oz.) water. Then turn heat down to medium and let simmer for another 20 - 25 minutes. Remove pot from heat to give amaranth a chance to swell some more, and if necessary, strain extra water through sieve.

How to Cook Quinoa

Before preparing them in any dish, quinoa grains need to be thoroughly rinsed under running water to rid them of their bitter substances. Then place quinoa in three times the amount of water - for example 200 g (7 oz.) quinoa in 600 ml (20 fl. oz.) water and bring to a boil. Then let swell for another 15 minutes at very low heat, either by turning the burner off, or, as in the old days, by wrapping the pot in a blanket and placing it under the eiderdown.

Caution!

The German Nutrition Society (DGE) strongly warns that infants below the age of 2 and people with intestinal inflammation should abstain from quinoa dishes!

Kaya: Coconut Jam (without egg)

Yields 1 jar

1 brown, ripe coconut

3 pandan leaves (or substitute with pandan essence, please see page 241, or buy at Asian market)

275 g (9.7 oz.) coconut flower sugar

1. Using the hammer and nail, make two good sized holes in the coconut shell. Drain coconut juice into a glass or porcelain receptacle.

2. Now, using hammer or saw (please work carefully!) crack coconut shell open and into pieces, then remove coconut meat from inside with a strong metal spoon. Cut larger parts into smaller pieces.

3. Along with half your saved coconut water, place coconut meat into blender and blend at highest speed for 4 minutes.

4. After covering an adequately large glass or porcelain bowl with a clean cheesecloth, place portions of coconut puree on it in steps. Over a second bowl press out coconut milk.

5. Pour coconut milk into a wok or deep non-stick frying pan. Tie knots in pandan leaves and, along with 200 g (7 oz.) sugar, add to milk in wok. Let come to a quick boil, then, whisking occasionally, let simmer until brown and creamy. This can take up to 50 minutes. Remove wok from heat and set aside.

6. To make caramel, heat 75 g (2.6 oz.) coconut blossom sugar in non-stick pan until it caramelizes and turns golden brown. Now place wok with coconut milk and sugar mixture back on low heat and slowly cook.

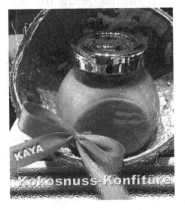

While cooking gently, slowly add caramelized sugar to wok. Wisk for another 5 -10 minutes until it turns golden brown with a creamy consistency.

7. Remove wok from heat and pandan leaves from Kaya cream. Once it has cooled off, blend in blender until it is silky smooth. Fill into sealable jars and refrigerate for up to 3 - 4 months.

Kaya: Coconut Jam (the original, with egg)
Yields one jar
5 eggs
½ cup coconut cream
¾ cup coconut milk
275 g (9.7 oz.) coconut blossom sugar
3 pandan leaves (substitute with pandan essence, please view page 241, or buy at Asian market)
1½ Tbsp. cooking starch

1. In a bowl, thoroughly whisk eggs, coconut milk and cream. (It goes faster with a mixer or in a blender, but whisking by hand makes the texture especially nice and smooth). Pour mixture into non-stick pan. Tie knots into pandan leaves and add to pan, or drizzle pandan essence into mixture. Slowly heat mass over medium heat and stir consistently with wooden spoon or using whisk, while gently letting mass cook. Do not boil, to keep eggs from setting.

2. Dissolve 1½ Tbsp. cooking starch in a little water and stir into kaya mass to thicken. Remove from heat and set aside.

3. To make caramel, heat 75 g (2.6 oz.) coconut blossom sugar in non-stick pan until it caramelizes and turns golden brown. Now place wok with coconut milk and sugar mixture back on low heat and slowly cook. Once it cooks gently, slowly add caramelized sugar to wok. Wisk for another 5 -10 minutes.

4. Remove wok from heat, and take pandan leaves out of Kaya cream. Once it has cooled off, blend in blender until it reaches a silky consistency. Fill into sealable jars. Refrigerated, kaya keeps for 7 - 9 days. Please do not eat once it smells sour or turns watery.

Tip: Also pandan leaves or pandan essence is not a must - but they do give this coconut jam its "certain exotic something".

For ultimate coconut aroma, you can purchase fresh coconut cream and milk from a company called "Kara". Your kaya will be lighter if you use only 50 g (1.7 oz.) of sugar. You can also make it with 4 or even only 3 eggs, but it will not be as creamy.

Gula-Malacca-Syrup

Yields about 40 ml (1.3 fl. oz.)

300ml (10.4 fl. oz.) non-carbonated water

10 pandan leaves (substitute with pandan essence, please view page 241, or buy at Asian market)

2 gula-malacca logs (or 200g/7 oz. coconut flower sugar).

1. Place gula-malacca logs into sauce pan with non-carbonated water. Tie knots into 6 of the pandan leaves and add to pan.
2. Bring to a boil over high heat, then lower heat and, stirring occasionally, let turn into a dark, thick syrup. This can take up to 1 hour. Remove pandan leaves after 20 minutes, adding the remaining 4 fresh ones to the syrup. These too, should be taken out after 20 minutes.
3. Stand a metal spoon in sealable glass jar to prevent it from cracking, then fill hot syrup into jar.

Gula-Malacca-syrup is the perfect refinement for ice cream and many desserts (for example Mimpi Manis, please see recipe below).

Mimpi Manis - Sweet Dream

Yields 2 servings

300 ml (10 fl. oz.) coconut milk (canned or homemade, please see page 237)

2½ Tbsp. dry chia seeds

1-1½ tsp. vanilla essence

1 fresh, very ripe mango

2 - 3 tsp. gula-malacca syrup (homemade, please see page 251)

If desired, coconut gratings and mint leaves for garnishing.

1. Stir chia seeds into glass or porcelain bowl with coconut milk and let swell in fridge for 30 minutes.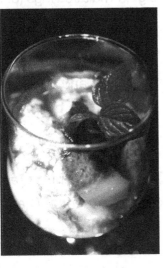

2. In the meantime, cut mango in two. To do so, on either side, make deep incisions, closely along the pit under the peel and turn halves in opposite directions to pry from pit. Next, cut mango flesh of each half lengthwise, down to the skin. Do not cut through skin. Now, to make mango cubes, cut criss-cross slices, again, down to the peel. Turn halves inside out and cut out popped up mango cubes with a knife. Also remove and slice mango flesh remaining on the sides of the pit.

3. Altering layers, now pour chia gel and mango cubes in tall, no too bulbous sundae glasses. Drizzle with gula-malacca and garnish with coconut gratings and mint leaves.

Tip: This dessert is also delicious with other types of fruit such as morello cherries (pitted), pineapple, kiwi or banana. To make frozen mimpi manis, freeze mango cubes for 30 - 45 minutes and/or splurge with a scoop of your favorite ice-cream.

Pumpkin-Spice Latte - the Original
Yields 1 large cup
9 Tbsp. coconut flower sugar
Seeds from 1 whole vanilla bean
300 ml (10 fl. oz.) water
1 cinnamon stick
2 dried star anise
½ tsp. freshly grated nutmeg
1 tsp. cinnamon powder
1 tsp. ground ginger
3 clove buds
3 allspice berries
1 pinch cardamom
1 sprinkling of ground Tonka bean (if so desired)
3 tsp. pumpkin mousse (please see page 254)
¼ l (8.4 fl. oz.) almond, coconut, quinoa, rice or oat milk
1 cup freshly brewed coffee
vegan cream, cinnamon or cocoa powder for garnishing

1. In a pot, bring 300 ml (10 fl. oz.) water, and sugar and vanilla to a boil. Lower heat to medium, add remaining spices and pumpkin mousse and, stirring occasionally, cook until you obtain a thick syrup.

2. Remove pot from heat and strain syrup through a coarse sieve, set aside to cool.
3. Heat up and froth nut milk in a pot. Fill into tall cup, adding as much syrup as you like. Top up with fresh coffee, garnish with vegan cream, sprinkle with cinnamon or cocoa powder. Enjoy hot!

Tip: When refrigerated, the remaining syrup sealed in a glass or porcelain container will keep for up to 6 months.

Quick Pumpkin-Spice Latte
Yields 1 large cup
3 tsp. coconut blossom sugar
2 tsp. pumpkin mousse
¼ l (8.4 fl. oz.) almond, coconut, quinoa, rice or oat milk
1 freshly brewed double espresso

1. In a tall cup, stir coconut flower sugar and 2 tsp. pumpkin mousse until smooth.
2. In a pot, boil and froth milk, and pour onto sugar-pumpkin mousse mixture.
3. Drizzle hot espresso in circular movements onto frothed milk. Enjoy hot!

Pumpkin Mousse
Pre-heat oven at 180 degrees (356 degrees Fahrenheit)
   Cut one small pumpkin Hokkaido into four pieces and remove seeds. Place pieces on baking tray laid out with baking parchment, and bake until pumpkin is soft.

Prick pumpkin meat with a fork to see if it is done. Scoop flesh out of shell with a sturdy spoon and purée in a blender until it reaches a creamy texture. If desired, you may add a little coconut oil. For either savory or sweet, flavor pumpkin mousse accordingly.

Matcha Tea Ice Cream (with egg yolk)
Yields up to 6 servings
200 ml (6.8 fl. oz.) vegan cream
3 - 4 tsp. matcha tea powder
350 ml (3.8 fl. oz.) almond, coconut, quinoa, rice or oat milk
100 g (3.5 oz.) coconut flower sugar
1 pinch of Himalaya salt
4 egg yolks

1. With a hand mixer, beat cream lightly and sprinkle on matcha tea powder. Keep beating at low speed until you have a bright green mass and all lumps are gone. Store in fridge.
2. Heat milk in a pan with sugar and the pinch of salt. Whisk until sugar has completely dissolved, remove from heat and set aside.
3. Whisk egg yolks in a bowl until they foam. Place pan with sugar-milk mixture back on heat, but only until it is on the verge of reaching boiling point.
4. While whisking constantly, slowly add egg yolks into heated mass. Do not boil or the eggs will curdle! While mixture simmers, keep whisking until it thickens. Then set aside.

5. Take matcha tea-cream out of fridge and very slowly add to thickened, hot yolk-milk mixture. Next, pour ice cream mass into ice cream maker and let the machine churn until ice cream is ready. Or, place finished match tea ice cream mass in glass or porcelain receptacle, or in a loaf baking pan laid out with parchment paper. Seal or cover well and freeze for at least 6 hours.

6. Scoop ice cream into tall glasses. Or remove ice cream from loaf pan and cut into slices and arrange on plates. Garnish servings with blackberries or raspberries and a waffle.

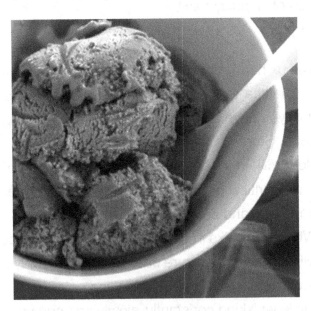

Matcha Tea Ice Cream (without egg yolk)

Yields up to 6 servings

4 tsp. matcha tea powder

½ l (2.1 cups) almond, coconut or oat milk

½ l (2.1 cups) vegan cream

180 g (6.3 oz.) coconut blossom sugar

1 pinch of Himalaya salt

Whisk all ingredients together until all sugar crystals are fully dissolved. Then either place in ice cream maker or freeze for 6 hours.

Quick and Easy Sorbet

For 2 servings

2 - 3 Tbsp. coconut flower sugar

100 g (3.5 oz.) Frozen fruit of your choice

1. Depending on your taste, stir 2 or 3 Tbsp. of coconut blossom sugar into 150 ml (5 fl. oz.) water until all sugar crystals fully dissolve.
2. Place frozen fruit in tall glass or porcelain container and drizzle with half the sugar water.
3. Blend with immersion blender until mixture reaches sorbet consistency. If needed, add more sugar water. Serve immediately!

Tip: To pep up your sorbet flavor, add some mint leaves, some lemon juice drops, or a splash of liqueur, or champagne, sparkling wine or prosecco.

Chia Recipes

Chia Muesli
Yields 1 serving
2 bananas, sliced
3 Tbsp. chia gel (please see page 246)
2 tsp. black raisins
1 Tbsp. unprocessed, lightly roasted pumpkin seeds

Peel banana and cut into average-size slices. In a bowl, combine and gently mix with chia gel, raisins and pumpkin seeds. Serve immediately.

Papabana Chia
For 1serving
1 banana
5 dried figs
200 g (7 oz.) papaya
5 tsp. ground chia seeds

1. Prepare this breakfast the night before. Peel and slice banana. Chop up figs and papaya flesh.
2. Combine prepared ingredients, and stir in chia seeds. Let swell overnight and enjoy the next morning.

Chia Lemon Salad Dressing
Yields 60 - 70 ml (2 - 2.4 fl. oz.)
1 lemon
2 Tbsp. dry chia seeds
1 - 2 Tbsp. coconut blossom sugar

1 Tbsp. Dijon mustard

2 - 3 Tbsp. coconut oil

According to taste, finely ground crystal, rock or pink Himalaya salt and black pepper from the mill.

1. Squeeze juice out of half a lemon. In a bowl, mix 4 Tbsp. lemon juice with sugar and whisk until crystals are fully dissolved.
2. Add Dijon mustard and coconut oil and whisk. Next, stir in chia seeds and blend until seeds have combined well with the liquid.
3. Cover and set dressing aside for 10 - 15 minutes, then, if you wish, add salt and pepper. Drizzle on salad and serve.

Chia Pan-Made Flat Bread

Yields about 4 servings

8 Tbsp. ground chia seeds

8 Tbsp. flour (for example quinoa, oat or spelt flour)

2 tsp. baking powder

2 eggs

½ grated onion (or substitute with ½ grated zucchini, or 1 large grated carrot)

1. In a large bowl, combine ground chia seeds, flour and baking powder and mix well.
2. Blend grated onion and eggs separately, then add to dry ingredients in first bowl. Blend well. Next, turn onto a lightly floured surface and knead until the dough is smooth.

3. Cut dough into four parts, then, with lightly moistened hands, form flat breads out of each one part.
4. In a non-stick frying pan, without fat, bake at medium heat for several minutes with the lid on. Serve flat bread hot.

Tip: To make hamburgers, simply slit bread in two halves. Place lettuce leaves, fried meat patty, tomato, pickle and cheese slices, along with onion rings on one half. Spread tomato sauce on the other half and use as top.

Chia Tutti-Frutti
Yields 1 serving
1 middle-seized apple (or 2 small apples)
8 pitted dates
1 Tbsp. dried goji berries
4 - 5 tsp. dried chia seeds

1. Chop apple and dates into small pieces. Combine with goji berries and chia seeds.
2. Set aside for 10 minutes to let flavors mix. Serve immediately.

Chia Almond Pudding
Yields up to 4 small servings
40 g (1.4 oz.) dry chia seeds
40 g (1.4 oz.) white almond butter (from organic food store)

1 Tbsp. ground ginger

1 tsp. vanilla powder

½ tsp. cinnamon powder

½ tsp. cardamom

300 ml (10 fl. oz.) water (or almond, quinoa or coconut milk instead)

3 Tbsp. coconut flower sugar (or 3 pitted dates)

1 pinch nutmeg

1. Combine all ingredients in blender and blend at highest speed until mass reaches creamy consistency.
2. Fill in small glass or porcelain bowls and chill in the fridge for at least 2 hours or over-night.

Chia Chocolate Pudding

For 1 serving

2 Tbsp. dry chia seeds

5 Tbsp. filtered water

1 tsp. Manuka honey

1 Tbsp. organic cocoa powder

1. Stir chia seeds into bowl with water and let swell for about 1 minute.
2. Next, add remaining ingredients and blend with immersion mixer. Fill into tall dessert glasses and chill for 15 minutes. Enjoy immediately!

Chia Applesauce

3 Tbsp. dry chia seeds

3 middle-sized apples

230 ml (7.8 fl. oz.) non-carbonated water

¼ tsp. cinnamon powder

1 splash lemon juice

coconut blossom sugar or Manuka honey to sweeten as desired

1. Grind chia seeds. Rinse, peel and core apples, and chop into small pieces.
2. Place apple pieces, water and cinnamon in a pot and bring to a boil. Turn heat to low and let cook gently for about 20 minutes. Spoon in water occasionally, if too much has evaporated from pot. Flavor with lemon juice, sugar or honey.
3. Combine apple mixture and chia seeds in blender and blend thoroughly. Fill applesauce in glass or porcelain dish and refrigerate for 1 hour.

Green Chia Kick

Yields 2 Glasses

4 dried plums

300 ml (10 fl. oz.) non-carbonated water

1 Tbsp. dry chia seeds

1 level tsp. matcha tea powder

1. Soak dried plums in non-carbonated water for 1 hour.

2. Remove plums from water and chop into small pieces. Use plum-soaking water to soak chia seeds and let swell for 10 minutes (this lets the seeds absorb the plum taste and nutrients).
3. Combine plum chunks with match tea powder and stir into chia gel. Cover mixture and set aside for 15 minutes. After that, fill green chia kick in a glass.

Chia Mango Coconut Ice Cream
Yields up to 4 servings
3 Tbsp. dry chia seeds
300 ml (10 fl. oz.) coconut milk
1 large, ripe mango
Optional: 2 - 3 Tbsp. lemon juice
Mango pieces and coconut gratings to garnish

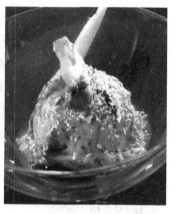

1. Stir chia seeds into coconut milk and let swell for 20 minutes. In the meantime, peel mango, separate flesh from pit and cut meat into small pieces.
2. Combine chia gel with coconut milk and mango pieces in blender and blend at highest speed.
3. Add lemon juice if you like, pour mass into ice cream maker and let churn. Or pour mixture into loaf-baking form laid out with baking parchment and freeze for 6 hours.
4. Scoop ice cream into glasses, or slice and serve on plates. Garnish with mango bits and coconut gratings.

Basic Chia Pancake Recipe

Yields 6 pancakes

4 Tbsp. chia gel (please view page?)

100 g (3.5 oz.) flour

150 ml (5 fl. oz.) non-carbonated water

Salt or sugar (depending on preference)

2 Tbsp. coconut oil.

1. Combine chia gel with 150 ml (5 fl. oz.) non-carbonated water and blend in blender or with immersion blender until it becomes a white liquid. If the mass gets too thick, add some more water.
2. Pour mass into new bowl, adding flour. You should obtain a kind of egg-pancake batter. For savory pancakes, add salt, or, for the sweet variety, sugar.
3. Heat oil in frying pan as needed. One at a time, fry up to 6 pancakes, flipping them on either side until golden brown.

Sweet Chia Pancakes

Mix basic chia pancake batter. Add 50 g (1.8 oz.) pitted and drained sour cherries (or any other fruit of your choice) into batter and flavor with coconut flower sugar. As described above, fry in coconut oil, and sprinkle finished pancakes with coconut flower sugar, or drizzle with Manuka honey. Garnish with cinnamon powder.

Tasty Chia Pancakes (savory)

Mix basic chia pancake batter and season with salt, pepper and a small, chopped garlic clove. Then fry, as described, 6 pancakes in coconut oil. When done, place slices of cheese and tomato and lettuce leaf and sprinkle some parsley on top. (Parsley can also go directly into batter before frying.)

Savory Chia Rolls

Yields 4 rolls

8 Tbsp. ground chia seeds

8 Tbsp. buckwheat flour (or quinoa, oat or spelt flour)

1 Tbsp. cooking starch

2 tsp. baking powder

2 eggs

½ grated onion

1. Pre-heat oven to 200 degrees (392 degrees Fahrenheit). In a bowl, combine ground chia seeds, flour and baking powder and mix well.
2. Mix eggs with grated onion and add to dry ingredients. Stir mixture thoroughly. Next, turn mass onto lightly floured surface and knead until dough is smooth.
3. Cut dough into four parts, forming rolls out of each one with slightly moistened hands. Slice a groove in each roll, not too deeply. Place rolls on floured baking pan and bake (on center rack) for 10 - 15 minutes.

Chia Cherry Jam (sweet or sour)

Yields 1 small jar

3 Tbsp. dry chia seeds

8 cherries (any kind of your choice)

50 ml (1.7 fl. oz.) cherry juice

¼ tsp. vanilla sugar

½ tsp. vanilla extract

Adding coconut blossom sugar or Manuka honey is optional

1. Grind up chia seeds. Pit cherries and blend coarsely in blender or with immersion blender
2. Combine cherry juice with vanilla sugar and extract along with fruit purée, blend and sweeten with sugar or honey, if so desired.
3. Add ground chia seeds and mix well. Fill jam into jar, not quite filling it to the top, since it will need some room to expand.
4. Refrigerate over-night and enjoy the next morning.

Tip: With this recipe, you can also make kiwi jam (1 ripe kiwi), orange jam (1/2 orange and some orange zest), plum jam (3 soft plums) or applesauce (1 apple).

Katharina's Chia Bread

Yields 1 loaf, approx. 700 g (24.7 oz.)

150 g (5.3 oz.) dry chia seeds (or chia seed flour)

400 g (14 fl. oz.) non-carbonated water

10 g (0.35 oz.) fresh yeast

1½ Tbsp. coconut blossom sugar

300 g (10.5 oz.) spelt, buckwheat or gluten-free flour (from organic food store)

10 - 12 g (0.28 - 0.42 oz.) fine rock, crystal or pink Himalaya salt

100 g (3.5 oz.) popped amaranth

Optional: 1¼ tsp. baking powder

1. Wait until all ingredients reach room temperature. Combine ground chia seeds or store-bought chia flour in blender with non-carbonated water and blend. Shape dough into ball, cover and set aside for 20 minutes.

2. In the meantime, in a cup, mix fresh yeast with 3 Tbsp. lukewarm water and ½ Tbsp. coconut flower sugar, stirring until sugar is dissolved. Cover cup and set aside in a warm place.

3. In a bowl, combine spelt, buckwheat or gluten-free flour with remaining sugar, salt and popped amaranth, and adding sieved baking powder, stir thoroughly. Spread 5 Tbsp. of flour mix onto work surface.

4. Place chia ball on top, and pour remaining dry ingredients on top of ball to form a small mound on work surface. Make a deep dent into the top of mound and pour in yeast-sugar mixture.

5. Next, working from the outer edges towards the middle, knead dry ingredients into dent, to form a

homogenous dough. Keep kneading for another 10 minutes. If it is still sticky, add some flour to hands and surface and work the dough some more.

6. Now roll dough into a ball, place in glass, porcelain or metal bowl at room temperature, cover with a dish towel and set aside to rest in a warm, draft-free place for 1 hour (or in oven at 40 degrees/104 degrees Fahrenheit).

7. When the hour is up, replace dough on floured surface and knead thoroughly for another 10 minutes. Then form into loaf shape, place on floured baking tray, cover with dish towel and let rest in a warm place again for a further hour, allowing loaf to rise. It should rise by one third of its size.

8. Pre-heat oven at 200 degrees (392 Fahrenheit) (please do not use convection setting in oven!). Place loaf on tray, lightly dust with flour and put in hot oven. Place small oven-proof bowl with water inside oven and bake loaf. After 20 minutes, lower heat to 180 degrees (356 Fahrenheit) and continue baking for another 60 minutes.

9. Towards the end, do the knock test: simply tap the top of loaf with a wooden spoon, or your knuckles. A hollow sound means the bread is done. If it sounds like more of a thud, it must go back in the oven.

Place bread loaf on oven grid to cool. Do not slice before it has cooled off. Store in fridge.

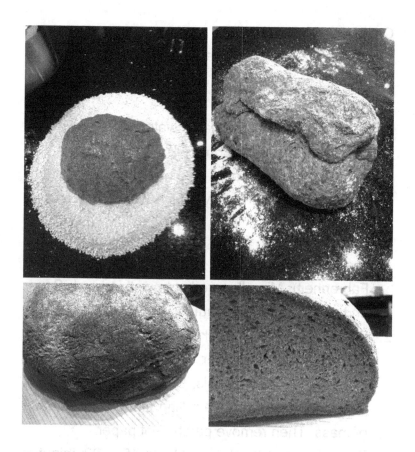

Tip: Refine chia bread recipe with 1 cup blanched carrot sticks, or roasted onions, pumpkin seeds or walnuts, garlic or dried tomato bits. Also chopped sultanas, dried plums or raisins are excellent to spruce up your flavor. Simply work chosen ingredients into dough during second kneading.

For savory bread, add 12 - 14 g (0.42 oz. - 0.49 0z.) salt. However, this bread does not go as well with sweet spreads or jams.

Chia Sesame Crackers

Yields up to 20 crackers, depending on size

1 Tbsp. dry chia seeds

1 Tbsp. sesame seeds

80 ml (3 fl. oz.) non-carbonated water

2 Tbsp. cold pressed coconut oil

¼ tsp. fine crystal, rock or pink Himalaya salt (or substitute with Tamari - soy sauce without gluten and wheat!)

1. Pre-heat oven to 170 - 180 degrees (325 - 356 Fahrenheit). Mix all ingredients well in bowl. Cover and set aside for 15 minutes.

2. Line baking tray with baking parchment and spread part of mass on paper as thinly and evenly as possible. To help with this, place second parchment paper on mass and use rolling pin to even surface of mass. Then remove parchment paper.

3. Bake in oven (center rack) for 15 - 20 minutes (your baking time depends on how thinly mass was spread), then remove from oven and gently un-stick half-baked mass from paper.

4. Using a pizza cutter, cut into squares and re-bake for another 15 minutes. Then flip crackers and add any of the following toppings below, then re-bake for another 5 - 10 minutes.

Spicy Cracker Topping

1 tsp. finely chopped onion

1 tsp. finely chopped tomato

1½ tsp. chili powder

½ tsp. cumin powder

½ tsp. sweet paprika powder

¼ tsp. fine crystal, rock or pink Himalaya salt.

Blend all ingredients well and sprinkle on crackers during last baking phase (please see above).

Chia Nut Cake

Yields 1 rectangular cake

1 large egg

6 large egg whites

2½ Tbsp. coconut flower sugar

2½ Tbsp. Manuka honey

3½ Tbsp. coconut oil

1 pinch tartar (from the pharmacy)

160 g (5.6 oz.) buckwheat flour

2 tsp. baking powder

50 g (1.8 oz.) walnuts

5 Tbsp. ground chia seeds

Drizzle with honey as icing, or dust with powdered sugar, as you like.

1. Pre-heat oven to 160 degrees (140 degrees Fahrenheit). With a hand-held mixer, blend 1 egg, 2 egg whites, half the sugar and honey to a creamy mass. Then, by the spoon, slowly add coconut oil.

2. Whisk remaining egg whites and sugar and pinch of tartar to a stiff texture.
3. Sift flour (minus 1 Tbsp.) and baking powder into separate bowl. Chop up walnuts in blender, adding 1 Tbsp. flour.
4. Taking turns, fold egg mixture and stiff egg whites respectively into sifted flour mixture. Next, stir in chopped walnuts and ground chia seeds.
5. Pour batter into greased baking pan and bake in oven (on center rack) for 40 minutes. Insert wooden toothpick to test if your cake is done. The wood should come out clean, without any batter streaks. Otherwise bake for another few minutes.
6. Tip cake out of pan onto baking grid and let cool. To coat, drizzle with honey or dust with powdered sugar.

Info: Pure tartar, also known as potassium tartrate, potassium bitartrate or calcium tartrate should not be confused with cream of tartar baking powder! In EU-countries, it is listed in the E category under number E336 (potassium tartrate in combination with potassium bitartrate) and under E354 (calcium tartrate), and is completely harmless for humans. Among other things, it is used to make caramel and tartaric acid, and stabilizes beaten egg whites and whipped cream. It also keeps sugar syrups from crystallizing. In pharmaceutical terms, it is called Lexans, known in the US as "cream of tartar".

Probably the Fastest Cupcake in the World
Yields 2 servings
6 Tbsp. ground chia seeds
1 egg
3 tsp. natural honey
1 level tsp. baking powder
1 tsp. coconut oil
1 Tbsp. cinnamon powder

1. Mix all ingredients together well. Pour into cups, glass or porcelain bowls or muffin pan, filling chosen containers only half way.
2. Bake batter for 70 seconds at 800 watts in a micro wave. Flip cakes on plates, sprinkle some coconut flakes (or other yummy ones) on top if you like, and Bingo, done!

Tip: This healthy treat tastes good for breakfast or as a quick afternoon snack for surprise guests. You can also pep up the batter with a few blueberries, dried cherries, walnuts or poppy seeds. Serve à la mode with a scoop of vanilla or lemon ice cream.

Chia Smoothie Tropicana
For 2 smoothies
2 tsp. dry chia seeds
180 ml (6 fl. oz.) coconut milk
1 peeled and deseeded orange
50 g (1.8 oz.) fresh, chopped pineapple

50 g (1.8 oz.) fresh, chopped mango

2 peeled bananas, cut into bits

180 ml (6 fl. oz.) non-carbonated water

Mint leaves for garnishing

1. Mix chia seeds into coconut milk and let swell for 10 minutes.
2. Blend prepared fruit in blender with non-carbonated water.
3. Fill blended fruit into two tall glasses and top up with coconut milk mixture. Stir and garnish with mint leaves.

Chia Lemon Drink

Yields 4 servings

90 ml (3 fl. oz.) freshly pressed lemon juice (or lime juice)

4 Tbsp. coconut blossom sugar

1.5 l (6.3 cups) non-carbonated water

2 Tbsp. dry chia seeds

Mint leaves optional

1. Fill glass carafe with lemon juice, sugar and water and stir well.
2. Add chia seeds and stir well again, making sure seeds are fully immersed in fluid. Add sugar if so desired, and let swell for 10 minutes.
3. Stir lemon-chia drink briefly before serving. Enjoy with ice cubes on hot days. Garnish carafe with mint leaves.

Chia Bubble Tea
Yields 2 servings
30 g (1 oz.) dry chia seeds
250 ml (8.4 fl. oz.) cold tea (any kind)
90 ml (3 fl. oz.) almond or coconut milk
coconut blossom syrup, natural honey or agave syrup
to sweeten
crushed ice to fill glasses

1. Stir chia seeds with tea and milk into carafe and let
   swell for 20 minutes.
2. Sweeten as much as you like and pour into tall
   glasses filled with crushed ice. Serve at once.

More Uses for Chia Seeds

Cauliflower Soup
Cook 1 large cauliflower (alternative: broccoli), save
water (500 ml or 16.8 fl. oz.) to bowl, spice to taste and
add 5 Tbsp. ground chia seeds. Blend well and serve
immediately.

Fun Potato Purée
Stir 2 Tbsp. of white and black chia seeds into prepared
potato purée

Tuna Fish Gel
Open tuna can without oil, drain water into bowl, adding
and stirring in 1 Tbsp. chia seeds. Let swell for 15

minutes. Spread tuna-gel and tuna meat on sandwich or roll and enjoy immediately.

Tuna Fish Paste
In a blender, combine tuna-gel with ½ can of tuna meat and spices to taste and blend vigorously. Enjoy paste on bread or roll.

Breadcrumbs Coating or its Substitutes
Combine 3 Tbsp. chia seeds, 2 Tbsp. almond flour and 2 tsp. garlic powder and spices to taste. Use as coating for fish, beef or chicken.

Baking Cakes and Cookies
Simply substitute half of flour amount from cake or cookie recipe with ground chia seeds.

Cheesecake Topping
Roast 3 Tbsp. ground chia seeds and mix in 4 tsp. honey and 1 tsp. cinnamon. Coat baked cheesecake with this mixture.

Puff Pastry
Thaw and roll out frozen puff pastry. Thoroughly mix 3 Tbsp. ground chia seeds with 4 Tbsp. honey, 1 tsp. cinnamon (and optionally 2 Tbsp. chopped walnuts). Spread on pastry and fold into turnovers. Bake according to package instructions.

Jellied Fruit for Tarts and Cakes
Mix 100 ml (3.4 fl. oz.) of fruit and fruit juice of your choice with 3 - 5 Tbsp. ground chia seeds. Let swell for 15 minutes and use gelled fruit as topping on cheesecake or as base in pie shell.

Sorbets
Pass fruit or berries of your choice through sieve, add some fruit juice (100 ml or 3.4 fl. oz.) and 3 Tbsp. chia seeds and mix well. Fill into container and freeze.

Energy Drink
Drain coconut water from coconut and mix with 2 Tbsp. chia seeds. Refrigerate for 15 minutes. This drink is energizing and especially hydrating on hot days.

Indian Lassi-Drink
In a blender, combine 1 Tbsp. chia seeds, 1 yoghurt and 100 ml (3.4 fl. oz.) of fruit juice of your choice and blend thoroughly. Serve in glasses.

Extended Nut Nougat Cream
Add 4 Tbsp. ground chia seeds to 1 jar of nut nougat cream, and you have a somewhat healthier sandwich spread.

Sago Starch Substitute
Ground chia seeds are ideal for thickening all types of fluids. The more seeds you use, the thicker the liquid gets. Find out by testing!

Amaranth Recipes

My Special Amaranth Muesli
For 1 serving
4 Tbsp. popped amaranth
2 Tbsp. plain yoghurt (from sheep or goat)
50 g (1.8 oz.) blueberries (or raspberries, or both)
1 tsp. natural honey or gula-malacca (please see page 251)
1 tsp. warmed up organic peanut butter
Combine all ingredients and serve immediately.

Amaranth-Pumpkin-Seed Patties
Yields 6 patties
1 large onion
3 garlic cloves
1 of each: small red, green and yellow pepper
1 small bunch fresh or 2 tsp. dried oregano
60 g (2.1 oz.) pumpkin seeds
1½ tsp. ground curcuma
6 - 8 Tbsp. coconut oil
250 g (8.8 oz.) ground amaranth
70 g (2.5 oz.) rice flour
200 g (7 oz.) organic soya protein
300 ml (10 fl. oz.) non-carbonated water
30 - 40 ml (1 - 1.3 fl. oz.) balsamic vinegar
20 - 30 ml (0.67 - 1 fl. oz.) Tamari (soy sauce without gluten and wheat!)
freshly ground black pepper from the mill
fine crystal, rock or pink Himalaya salt to taste

1. Peel and finely chop onion and garlic. Rinse, clean and cube peppers. Rinse fresh oregano and shake dry. Remove leaves from stem and chop.
2. In a pan without fat, roast pumpkin seeds and curcuma at high temperature. Set aside in small bowl. Place 1 Tbsp. coconut oil in pan to fry onions, garlic and pepper cubes.
3. In a new bowl, combine amaranth, rice flour, Tamari, protein and approx. 200 ml (6.8 fl. oz.) water. Add pumpkin seeds and curcuma and blend well. Should the mass be too dry, add some water.
4. Flavor with balsamic vinegar, Tamari sauce and black pepper from the mill. Add salt if necessary.
5. With lightly moistened hands, form small balls out of mass. Heat remaining coconut oil, place balls in pan, carefully flattening them with a spoon to form round patties. These should be about 2 cm (0.8 in) thick. Try to keep edges from fraying too much. Fry on both sides, till brown and crunchy. Serve amaranth-pumpkin patties with salads, veggies or grilled salmon.

Savory Amaranth-Cheese Patties
Yields approx. 12 patties
For coating you need:
4 Tbsp. coconut flour
6 Tbsp. spelt bread crumbs

For patties:

300 ml (10 fl. oz.) hearty vegetable broth (prepare hearty broth)

140 g (4.9 oz.) amaranth

2 onions

2 garlic cloves

1 bunch fresh parsley

4 Tbsp. chopped pumpkin seeds (or chopped hazelnut instead)

3 eggs (or chia-egg substitute, please see page 246)

60 gr. popped amaranth (or substitute with 4 Tbsp. spelt bread crumbs)

5 Tbsp. hard cheese, grated

2 tsp. Dijon mustard

½ tsp. crystal, rock or pink Himalaya salt (or substitute with Tamari - soy sauce without gluten and wheat!)

5 Tbsp. coconut oil for frying

4 Tbsp. spelt bread crumbs

1. Combine all ingredients for breading.
2. Fill veggie broth in pot, adding amaranth and bring to a boil. Reduce temperature, cover with lid and let cook gently for another 25 minutes. Then, remove from heat and set aside to cool. Drain any excess fluid from pot.
3. While amaranth is cooking, peel and cube onions and garlic. Rinse parsley and shake dry, finely chop leaves. Chop up pumpkin seeds.

4. In a large bowl, combine cooled off amaranth with onions, garlic, eggs, pumpkin seeds, popped amaranth, grated cheese, chopped parsley and mustard and blend well, adding salt and pepper as desired.

5. Shape patties out of mass and roll in bread crumb coating. Heat coconut in pan and fry on both sides until brown and crunchy. Tastes good when served with salad with chia-lemon dressing (please see page 258).

Tip: As an alternative coating, use only whole grain bread crumbs.

Instead of amaranth, you may also use the same amount of quinoa. Please remember to rinse quinoa thoroughly before cooking.

Amaranth Waffles
50 g (1.8 oz.) whole grain flour (or other flour of your choice)
1 tsp. baking powder
½ tsp. starch
½ tsp. cinnamon or vanilla powder
150 ml (5 fl. oz.) almond, quinoa or rice milk
30 g (1 oz.) coconut flower sugar
50 g (1.8 oz.) popped amaranth

1. Pre-heat waffle maker to desired temperature. In the meantime, combine flour, baking powder, starch and cinnamon or vanilla powder in large bowl.

2. Add milk and sugar and whisk to a smooth batter, removing all lumps.
3. Add popped amaranth and blend in carefully. Ladle batter in and bake waffles until golden brown. Serve waffles adding thin layer of kaya (coconut jam, please see page 247). Or top with fresh fruit, such as strawberries, blueberries, sliced apple and/or à la mode with ice-cream of your choice.

Sweet Poppi Candy
Yields 3 - 4 pieces
3 Tbsp. popped amaranth
1 Tbsp. natural honey
1 Tbsp. organic peanut butter
1 Tbsp. coconut oil

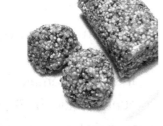

1. Blend all ingredients together well
2. Spread mass on baking parchment and shape into ball, rounds or squares, as you like. Rap each ball, round or square in parchment paper and refrigerate for 2 hours for them to set. Enjoy!

Qunioa Recipes

Quinoa Purée
Boil ½ l (2.1 cups) water. Stir in 180 - 230 g (6.3 - 8 oz.) quinoa flakes and whisk until you have quinoa purée. Quickly remove from heat and flavor with crystal, rock

or pink Himalaya salt, some coconut oil and a dash of nutmeg powder. (It needs a little stronger flavoring than normal potato purée - please test to find out.)

Quinoa and Mixed Vegetable Dish
Yields 2 Servings
200 g (7 oz.) mixed quinoa (red, white, and black)
600 ml (20 fl. oz.) hearty veggie broth
1 large onion
2 garlic cloves
1 of each: large red, green and yellow pepper
1 Tbsp. coconut oil
crystal, rock or pink Himalaya salt (or substitute with Tamari - soy sauce without gluten and wheat!)

1. Rinse quinoa thoroughly, place into pan with veggie broth and bring to a boil. Slowly cook at medium heat for 20 - 25 minutes. Then remove from heat and set aside for 15 minutes.
2. In the meantime, peel and cube onions and garlic. Rinse, clean and cube peppers.
3. Drain quinoa through sieve. Heat 1 Tbsp. coconut oil in frying pan. First add garlic, then onions, and peppers last, and sauté for 1 - 2 minutes. Stir briefly and add quinoa. Mix well and fry for another 10 minutes. Flavor with pink Himalaya salt or Tamari to taste.

Quinoa Patties in Spicy Sauce

Yields up to 12 patties

For sauce:

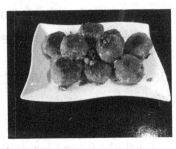

1 large onion

2 garlic cloves

1 red bell pepper

1 small chili pepper

200 g (7 oz.) fresh button mushrooms

1 Tbsp. coconut oil

150 g (5.3 oz.) fresh corn

3 Tbsp. tomato paste

150 ml (5 fl. oz.) veggie broth

crystal, rock, or pink Himalaya salt

white pepper

Tabasco

red curry paste

sweet paprika powder

vegan crème fraîche

For the patties:

200 g (7 oz.) quinoa

1 small leek

600 ml (20 fl. oz.) veggie broth

1 tsp. fine crystal, rock, or pink Himalaya salt

½ - 1 large onion

4 - 5 Tbsp. coconut oil

2 eggs (or chia egg substitute, see page 246)

3 Tbsp. millet flakes

whole grain breadcrumbs (or amaranth loaf breadcrumbs)

1. Peel and finely cube onion and garlic. Clean and wash bell pepper, and chili pepper and rub mushrooms clean. Chop into small cubes.

2. Heat coconut oil in pan, sauté onion and garlic, next add bell and chili peppers, and mushrooms and sauté also.

3. Stir in corn, tomato paste and veggie broth. Flavor with salt, pepper, Tabasco, curry paste and paprika powder. Last, stir in crème fraîche, set aside and keep sauce warm.

4. To make the patties, wash quinoa and leek thoroughly. Let broth with quinoa and salt come to a boil, then reduce heat to medium and let cook gently for another 20 - 25 minutes. Remove from heat and set aside for 15 minutes.

5. In the meantime, peel and cube onion and cut leek in thin rings.

6. Heat up 1 Tbsp. coconut oil in a pan, add onions and leek and fry. Next, place quinoa in a large bowl, adding fried onions and leek.

7. Mix eggs and millet flakes and stir until mass is homogenous. (Add millet in steps, the mass should be malleable, but not too dry). Form patties with moistened hands, and roll in breadcrumbs if desired.

8. Heat up remaining coconut oil in pan and fry patties on both sides until brown and crisp. Serve with spicy sauce, salad or vegetables.

Quinoa Coconut Dessert

Yields 4 servings

200 g (7 oz.) quinoa

4 small, aromatic apples

3 Tbsp. grapes

400 ml (14 fl. oz.) coconut milk (or almond, quinoa or oat milk

1 pinch crystal, rock, or pink Himalaya salt

1 Tbsp. coconut butter

3 Tbsp. chopped almonds

1 tsp. cinnamon powder

sweeten to taste with either coconut blossom sugar or nectar, Manuka honey or natural agave syrup, coconut gratings

1. Rinse quinoa, apples and grapes well. Peel apples, core and cut in little pieces.
2. Combine milk, quinoa, butter and salt in sauce pan and bring to a boil.
3. Add and stir apple bits, almonds, grapes and cinnamon into mixture, and let simmer at low temperature for 25 minutes.
4. Remove from heat and sweeten to taste. Before serving, sprinkle with coconut gratings.

Tip: On Fun Days (please see page 24, all about "Fun Day Rule"), add whipped vegan cream, carefully folding into quinoa coconut dessert.

Fun Day Recipes

Baby Potatoes
Yields 4 servings
15 small potatoes
1 large onion
one of each: red, green and yellow bell peppers
2 - 3 garlic cloves
2 Tbsp. coconut oil
1 pinch crystal, rock or pink Himalaya salt
freshly ground black pepper from the mill

1. Wash potatoes and bell peppers. Boil unpeeled potatoes until soft, drain water and set aside to cool off. Next, leaving on peel, cut into thin slices.
2. Clean out peppers and cube, peel and cube onion and garlic cloves. Heat up coconut oil in pan, then add peppers, onion and garlic and sauté.
3. Add potato slices and fry lightly. Stir and season with salt and pepper. Serve with salad of choice and/or with chicken breast or beef filet, fried in coconut oil.

Heavenly Coconut Cupcakes, with White Chocolate-Matcha-Mint Buttercream

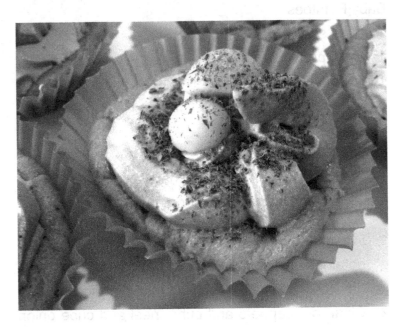

Yields 12 cupcakes

For the batter:

180 ml (6 fl. oz.) coconut milk

3 large egg whites (or chia egg substitute, please see page 246)

130 g (4.5 oz.) wheat flour (or other flour of choice)

3 Tbsp. coconut blossom sugar

2 heaping tsp. baking powder

¼ tsp fine crystal, rock or pink Himalaya salt

80 g (2.8 oz.) butter at room temperature

if desired, either 50 g (1.8 oz.) peeled walnut halves, or 50 g (1.8 oz.) finely chopped walnuts

For the buttercream:

1 bar of white chocolate

1 Tbsp. coconut flower sugar

4 Tbsp. non-carbonated water

2 large egg whites (these cannot be replaced by chia seeds!)

150 g (5.3 oz.) butter at room temperature, yet not too soft

2 heaping tsp. matcha tea powder

2 - 3 drops peppermint oil (more, if you like it really minty.)

1. Pre-heat oven to 180 degrees (356 Fahrenheit). Place muffin pan, or cupcake cups, or 12 oven-proof bowls on center rack or baking tray.

2. To make batter, in a small bowl, beat coconut milk and egg whites (here you may use chia seed egg substitute). In a second bowl, sift together flour, sugar, salt, and baking powder.

3. Add coconut milk mixture and butter to flour mixture and whisk until you have a smooth batter. Scoop batter into pre-heated muffin tins, filling them just two thirds.

4. Bake for 25 minutes, then prick muffin with tooth pick. If it comes out clean with no batter sticking to it, cupcakes are done. If not, bake for another few more minutes. Pop muffins out of pan and set on rack to cool.

5. To make buttercream, melt white chocolate in water bath and set aside.

6. Heat up water and sugar in a sauce pan. Do not stir, swivel pot gently instead, the sugar should not caramelize. After 2 minutes, remove pot from heat.
7. Whisk egg whites until stiff with a hand held mixer. Next, while constantly beating (at lowest speed), slowly pour sugar solution in, down inside edge of bowl. Keep whisking until egg white has cooled.
8. Next, add butter in by the spoon. Stir slowly, until you get buttercream consistency. Mix matcha tea powder and peppermint oil into melted white chocolate, then carefully work this mixture into buttercream.
9. Fill buttercream into piping bag with nozzle. (If the buttercream is too soft, place in fridge for a few minutes). Decorate cupcakes with buttercream and top with walnut halves or chopped walnuts.

Tip: Instead of wheat flour, you can grind up amaranth to flour and mix with spelt or rye flour at a ratio of 1:2.

When the butter for buttercream is too cold, it tends to clump. To avoid clumping, simply beat butter at higher speed until smooth. When the butter is too soft, the mass can be too liquid. In this case, add some cold butter to harden again.

After Eight Ice Cube Chocolates
Yields about 20 pieces
100 g (3.5 oz.) powdered sugar
approx. 2 - 3 tsp. non-carbonated water

1 tsp. peppermint oil (or more if you like)

2 bars of dark chocolate (70% cocoa content)

1 Tbsp. coconut oil

1. Stir powdered sugar into water until you get thick, moist mass. Add water by the teaspoon! If the mass is too liquid, add a little sugar. Work in peppermint oil to taste. Refrigerate to chill over-night.

2. Next day, place white chocolate and coconut oil in water bath and melt (no hotter than 35 degrees, or 95 Fahrenheit). Remove from heat.

3. Place small candy cups on baking tray. Fill with melted chocolate, just covering the bottom. Take peppermint mixture from fridge and stir briefly. Fill ¼ tsp. into each candy cup. Next, set aside to cool for about 1 hour. Finally, top up with melted chocolate, set aside to cool for 2 hours and only then refrigerate for 3 hours to harden thoroughly.

Tip: Instead of store-bought chocolate, you can use the homemade version made of cocoa powder and coconut oil (please see recipe below).

Coconut Ice Cube Chocolates

Yields up to 20 pieces

100 g (3.5 oz.) coconut blossom sugar

1½ cups non-carbonated water

90 g (3.2 oz.) cold pressed coconut oil

60 g (2.1 oz.) real cocoa powder (or cocoa beans)

1. Bring water and sugar to a boil in a pot. Let simmer over low to medium heat until syrupy. Then remove from heat.
2. In a second pot, heat up coconut oil to a maximum of 35 degrees (95 Fahrenheit) (check with kitchen thermometer). Add cocoa powder to oil and, using metal whisk, whisk until smooth.
3. Sweeten chocolate mass with coconut syrup to taste. Fill into candy cups and let cool for 2 hours. Finally, refrigerate for 3 hours.

Tip: I recommend cocoa powder made of Criollo cocoa beans in raw quality, or real "Domori" or "Caotina Surfin" cocoa powder. Or simply melt (just like for the After Eight Ice Cube Chocolates) chocolate with 70% cocoa content in water bath, adding in oil and syrup. Coconut oil may also be replaced by cocoa butter.

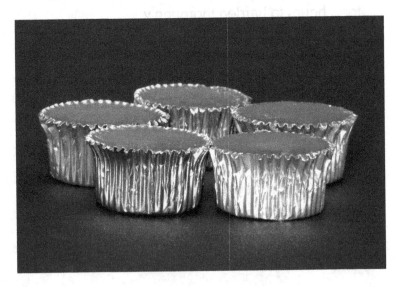

I'd love to read all about your experiences and ideas for recipes. Just email me at Info@katharinabachman.de

Unusual Creations by Berlin - Restaurant Owner Alfons Breiers

On my lecture tours with AIDA Cruises, I meet all kinds of people. One day, Alfons Breiers and his wife Bärbel appeared next to the stage, wanting to speak with me. We had a wonderful afternoon, which opened a whole new world of information on healthy foods. As a child, Alfons grew up with and was intrigued by herbs. In 2003, he opened the first restaurant in Rathsdorf, a village near Berlin, specializing in healthy, natural eating. Characteristic for his menu creations are the countless edible flowers and 260 different healthy, beneficial herbs. But also his classic dishes are palate-pleasing. He was kind enough to let me share three of his special recipes:

Homemade Mayonnaise
Yields approx. 250 - 300 g (8.8 - 10.5 oz.) mayonnaise
100 g (3.5 oz.) cashew nuts or almonds
100 g (3.5 oz.) non-carbonated water
12 g (0.4 oz.) mustard
50 g (1.8 oz.) vinegar
2 tsp. pink Himalaya salt
2 tsp. honey
good-seized pinch curcuma

250 g (8.8 oz.) coconut oil (or sunflower seed oil, or peanut oil)

1. Combine all ingredients except oil in strong blender and blend.
2. Next, slowly mix in oil and flavor mayonnaise again to taste. Store in fridge.

Tip: When using coconut oil to make mayonnaise, be sure it is at room temperature. If you store it in fridge, it will be hardened. It is best to remove from fridge 2 hours beforehand or to liquefy oil in a water bath.

Vegan Bolognaise Sauce
Yields 4 servings
2 Tbsp. sunflowers seeds
2 Tbsp. pumpkin seeds
200 ml (6.8 fl. oz.) non-carbonated water
½ onion
1 - 2 garlic cloves
2 Tbsp. coconut oil
4 fresh tomatoes
½ red bell pepper
6 sun-dried tomatoes
1 bunch basil
crystal, rock or Himalaya salt
pepper
nutmeg
1 - 2 Tbsp. agave syrup

1. Soak sunflower and pumpkin seeds in non-carbonated water for 2 hours.
2. Peel and finely chop onions and garlic and sauté in a pan with coconut oil.
3. Wash fresh tomatoes and bell pepper and coarsely chop along with sun-dried tomatoes. Rinse basil, shake dry and remove leaves from stems.
4. Fill tomatoes, bell pepper, onion and garlic and basil in blender. Adding salt, pepper, nutmeg and agave syrup, blend to a thick sauce.
5. Strain soaked sunflower and pumpkin seeds through sieve and chop coarsely. Work into sauce and season again if necessary. Mix sauce into hot spaghetti (cooked according to package instructions) and serve immediately.

Tip: This sauce is excellent with raw vegetable pasta. Wash cucumber or zucchini and scoop out seeds with a spoon. Slice veggie in long, thin strips and mix with sauce.

Mocha Balls
Yields approx. 20 balls
37 g (1.3 oz.) cocoa beans
22 g (0.8 oz.) cashew nuts or almonds
1 cm (0.4 inches) of a vanilla bean
3 g (0.10 oz.) coffee beans
22 g (0.8 oz.) honey
10 g (0.35 oz.) coconut flower sugar
10 g (0.35 oz.) cocoa liqueur

1 good seized pinch cinnamon powder
cocoa powder and coconut blossom sugar for coating

1. In a blender, finely chop, nuts, vanilla bean, coffee and cocoa beans.
2. Next, add honey, sugar, liqueur and cinnamon powder and keep blending until mixture is smooth. Shape little balls and roll in cocoa powder or coconut flower sugar for coating. Store in fridge.

Tip: You can find cocoa and coffee bean nibs, as well as cocoa liqueur, to buy on the internet.

If you would like to know more about Alfons Breiers and his timber-frame-style restaurant, please visit his family business website at: www.breiers-kraeutergarten.de

Lastly …

Dear reader,

Perhaps one day, even despite my healthy diet and all the wonderful substances and ingredients nature offers me on a daily basis, I will suddenly drop dead prematurely. Who's to know? Perhaps our death is predetermined exactly and there's not a thing we can do about it. But this I can tell you in all certainty: healthy eating and all that that entails, has filled my life with immeasurable joy, not to mention the return of a wonderful sense of well-being in my body. That alone, made it all worth it! And, incidentally, according to Confucius, a road was made for the journey, not the destination.

So, should I reach the age of a hundred, I will be back to tell more of the story. Or, in the meantime, you can visit my video-blog at www.sos-exercise-schmexercise.com or www.KatharinaBachman.de which I hope you will find very enjoyable.

Katharina Bachman

Coming soon ...

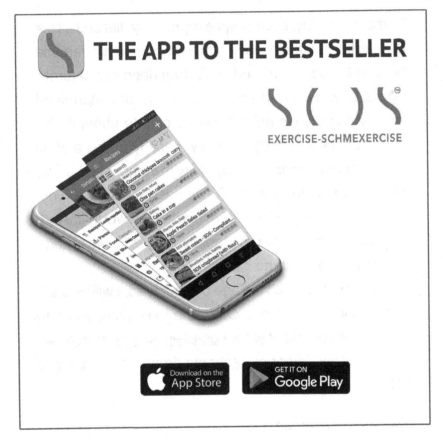
Please stay tuned and ask for News:

Info@sos-exercise-schmexercise.com

Sugar Content

per 100 g (3.5 oz.) (fresh not dried)	Fruit Sugar Fructose/Gram	Glucose/Gram
Rhubarb	0.39 (0.013 oz.)	0.41 (0.014 oz.)
Mango	2.60 (0.091 oz.)	0.85 (0.029 oz.)
Dragon Fruit	0.12 (0.004 oz.)	1.28 (0.045 oz.)
Papaya	0.34 (0.011 oz.)	1.03 (0.036 oz.)
Peach	1.24 (0.043 oz.)	1.04 (0.036 oz.)
Clementine	1.69 (0.059 oz.)	1.53 (0.053 oz.)
Pear	6.75 (0.23 oz.)	1.67 (0.058 oz.)
Mandarin	1.30 (0.045 oz.)	1.70 (0.059 oz.)
Apricot	0.86 (0.030 oz.)	1.73 (0.061 oz.)
Nectarine	1.79 (0.06 oz.)	1.79 (0.063 oz.)
Honeydew	3.91 (0.13 oz.)	2.02 (0.071 oz.)
Apple	5.74 (0.20 oz.)	2.04 (0.071 oz.)
Strawberry	2.28 (0.08 oz.)	2.16 (0.076 oz.)
Pineapple	2.59 (0.091 oz.)	2.26 (0.079 oz.)
Orange	2.58 (0.091 oz.)	2.27 (0.080 oz.)
Guava	2.75 (0.097 oz.)	2.35 (0.082 oz.)
Quince	4.29 (0.15 oz.)	2.67 (0.094 oz.)
Grapefruit	2.53 (0.089 oz.)	2.87 (0.101 oz.)
Watermelon	2.90 (0.10 oz.)	2.90 (0.102 oz.)
Plum	2.02 (0.071 oz.)	3.38 (0.119 oz.)
Lemon	3.45 (0.12 oz.)	3.58 (0.126 oz.)
Gooseberry	4.02 (0.14 oz.)	3.63 (0.128 oz.)
Banana	3.64 (0.12 oz.)	3.79 (0.133 oz.)
Damask Plum	2.00 (0.070 oz.)	4.30 (0.015 oz.)
Kiwi	4.41 (0.155 oz.)	4.71 (0.166 oz.)
Lychee	3.40 (0.11 oz.)	5.10 (0.179 oz.)
Yellow Plum	4.30 (0.151 oz.)	5.10 (0.179 oz.)
Passion Fruit	3.96 (0.13 oz.)	5.13 (0.180 oz.)
Sour Cherry	4.28 (0.15 oz.)	5.18 (0.182 oz.)
Sweet Cherry	6.14 (0.21 oz.)	6.93 (0.244 oz.)
Fig	5.51 (0.19 oz.)	6.99 (0.246 oz.)
Berry Fruit	7.63 (0.26 oz.)	7.33 (0.258 oz.)
Grapes (light)	7.63 (0.26 oz.)	7.33 (0.258 oz.)
Grapes (red)	7.63 (0.26 oz.)	7.93 (0.279 oz.)
Rose Hip	8.69 (0.30 oz.)	8.70 (0.306 oz.)
Date	31.33 (1.10 oz.)	33.60 (1.185 oz.)

Nutritional Values

Nutritional Values	White Sugar	Brown Sugar	Sugar Cane Sugar	Coconut Flower Sugar
Quantity	100 g (3.5 oz.)	100 g (3.5 oz.)	100 g (3.5 oz.)	100 g (3.5 oz.)
Energy	1619 J	1577 J	1632 J	1625 J
Energy	387 Cal	377 Cal	390 Cal	378,9 Cal
Protein	0 g	0 g	0 g	1.2 g
Carbohydrates	99.98 g	97.33 g	97.4 g	93.4 g
Fat	0 g	0 g	0 g	1.0 g
Sat. Fatty Acid	0 g	0 g	0 g	0.5 g
Fiber	-	-	-	2.2 g
Sodium	-	39 mg	-	90 mg
Potassium	0.2 mg	346 mg	-	1.011 mg
Calcium	0 g	0 g	0 g	1.5 mg
Protein	0 g	0 g	0 g	10 mg
Magnesium	0 g	0 g	0 g	31 mg
Iron	0 g	0 g	0 g	1.8 mg
Zinc	0 g	0 g	0 g	1.9 mg
Vitamin B1	0 g	0 g	0 g	73 mg
Vitamin B3	0 g	0 g	0 g	38.21 mg
Vitamin B6	0 g	0 g	0 g	33.29 mg
Vitamin C	0 g	0 g	0 g	20.1 mg
Humidity Content	0 g	0 g	0 g	2.52 %

100 grams (3.5 oz.) Chia Seeds Contain as Much... (p.309)

- Iron as 400 g (14 oz.) spinach
- Calcium as 500 ml (16.8 fl. oz.) milk
- Omega-3-Fatty Acid as 1kg (2.2 lbs.) salmon
- Fiber as 400 g (14 oz.) linseed
- Antioxidants as 900 g (1.98 lbs.) oranges

Nutritional Values	Chia Seeds
	Per 100 g
Energy	2194 J
	524 Cal
Total Fat Content	31.4 g
Saturated Fatty Acids	4.0 g
Monounsaturated Fats	2.1 g
Omega-6 Fatty Acids	6.4 g

Omega-3 Fatty Acids	20.4 g
Trans-Fatty Acids	0 g
Cholesterol	0 g
Total Fiber	33.7 g
Soluble Fiber	4 g
Insoluble Fiber	29.7 g
Protein	21.2 g

Chia Seeds per 100 g	Contain	2 Tbsp. Cover Daily Requirement	Recommended Daily Requirement
Vitamin B1	0.89 mg	18%	
Vitamin B3, Niacin	11.2 mg	17%	
Vitamin E	29.1 mg	50%	
Boron	0.03 mg		
Calcium	500 mg		10%
Iron	6.5 mg		10%
Potassium	600 mg		6%
Copper	1.5 mg		20%
Magnesium	290 mg		20%
Phosphorus	535 mg		16%
Selenium	< 0.2 mg		-
Zinc	5 mg		14%
Sodium	< 0.01 g		

	Amaranth	Quinoa	Corn	Millet	Oat
Nutritional Value	Per 100 g	Per 100 g	Per 100 g	Per 100 g	Per 100 g
Energy	1565 J	1565 J	360 J	494 J	1628 J
	374 Cal	374 Cal	86 Cal	118 Cal	389 Cal
Protein	14.45 g	13.1 g	3.22 g	3.5 g	16.89 g
Carbohydrates	66.17 g	68.9 g	19.02 g	23.57 g	66.27 g
Fat	6.51 g	5.8 g	1.18 g	1 g	6.9 g
Sugar	0 g	0 g	3.22 g	0.13 g	0 g
Saturated Fats	1.662 g	0.59 g	0.182 g	0.171 g	1.217 g
Monounsaturated Fats	1.433 g	1.535 g	0.347 g	0.183 g	2.178 g
Polyunsaturated Fats	2.891 g	2.347 g	0.559 g	0.506 g	2.535 g
Cholesterol	0 g	0 g	0 g	0 g	0 g
Fiber	9.3 g	5.9 g	2.7 g	1.3 g	10.6 g

Sodium	0.021 g	0.021 g	0.015 g	0.168 g	0.002 g
Potassium	0.366 g	0.740 g	0.270 g	0.062 g	0.429 g

Caloric Analysis:	%	%	%	%	%
Carbohydrates	72	75	76	80	70
Protein	13	12	13	12	15
Fat	15	13	11	8	15

	Rice Cooked	White Rice Cooked	Whole Grain Rice Cooked	Jasmin Rice	Brown Rice	Brown Rice Cooked
Nutritional Values	Per 100 g	Per 100 g	Per 100 g	Per 100 g	Per 100 g	Per 100 g
Energy	544 J	544 J	469 J	1456 J	460 J	464 J
	130 Cal	130 Cal	112 Cal	348 Cal	110 Cal	111 Cal
Protein	2.36 g	2.38 g	2.32 g	6.8 g	2.56 g	2.58 g
Carbohydrates	28.73 g	28.59 g	23.51 g	80 g	22.78 g	22.96 g
Fat	0.19 g	0.21 g	0.83 g	0 g	0.89 g	0.9 g
Sugar	0 g	0 g	0 g	0 g	0.35 g	0.35 g
Saturated Fats	0.051 g	0.065 g	0.165 g	0 g	0.179 g	0.18 g
Monounsaturated Fats	0.058 g	0.121 g	0.3 g	0 g	0.325 g	0.327 g
Polyunsaturated Fats	0.05 g	0.056 g	0.296 g	0 g	0.321 g	0.323 g
Cholesterol	0 g	0 g	0 g	0 g	0 g	0 g
Fiber	0 g	0.3 g	1.8 g	0.4 g	1.8 g	1.8 g
Sodium	0 g	0 g	0.001 g	0 g	0.301 g	0.005 g
Potassium	0.026 g	0.029 g	0.079 g	0 g	0.043 g	0.043 g

Caloric Analysis:	%	%	%	%	%	%
Carbohydrates	92	91	86	92	83	85
Protein	7	8	8	8	10	8
Fat	1	1	6	0	7	7

	Potato, Raw	Potatoes	Pasta	Pasta	Whole-Grain Pasta	Whole-Grain Pasta
	2.16 – 2.95 in.	Cooked, salted	Cooked	Dry	Dry	Cooked
Nutritional Value	Diameter	Per 100g (3.5 oz.)	Per 100g (3.5 oz.)	Per 100g (3.5 oz.)	Per 100g (3.5 oz.)	Per 100g (3.5 oz.)
Energy	490 J	346 J	657 J	1552 J	1456 J	519 J
	117 Cal	87 Cal	157 Cal	371 Cal	348 Cal	124 Cal
Protein	2.81 g	1.87 g	5.76 g	13.04 g	14.63 g	5.33 g
Carbohydrates	26.24 g	20.13 g	30.68 g	74.67 g	75.03 g	26.54 g
Fat	0.17 g	0.87 g	0.92 g	1.51 g	1.4 g	0.54 g
Sugar	1.92 g	0.87 g	0.56 g	1.77 g	0 g	0.8 g
Saturated Fat	0.043 g	0.1 g	0.175 g	0.277 g	0.258 g	0.099 g
Monounsaturated Fats	0.003 g	0.002 g	0.13 g	0.171 g	0.195 g	0.075 g
Polyunsaturated Fats	0.07 g	0.043 g	0.317 g	0.564 g	0.556 g	0.213 g
Cholesterol	0 g	0 g	0 g	0 g	0 g	0 g
Fiber	4 g	2 g	1.8 g	3.2 g	0 g	4.5 g
Sodium	0.010 g	0.240 g	0.232 g	0.005 g	0.008 g	0.003 g
Potassium	0.680 g	0.379 g	0.045 g	0.162 g	0.215 g	0.044 g

Caloric Analysis:	%	%	%	%	%	%
Carbohydrates	89	93	80	83	81	81
Protein	10	6	15	14	16	15
Fat	1	1	5	3	3	4

Afterword

I am by no means promoting any of the products mentioned in this book, nor do I receive any kind of compensation in money or gift form, nor do I benefit in any other way. I mention them exclusively as part of my personal life experience. With this in mind, I would like to mention that not all labels reading "organic" are necessarily what they claim to be. Nor, on the other hand, are products not labeled as such necessarily bad either. Therefore, find out, to the best of your ability, where the product comes from and was produced, and according to which rules and regulations, and under which circumstances it was brought to the store shelf.

I have written this by my own rule that "If you can't explain it clearly and in words anyone can understand, don't bother". I tried to de-mystify terms and concepts from medicine, biology, physics and science that sound exotic to most of us laypeople. I hope I have succeeded.

Doctor. K.S., whom I have repeatedly mentioned here, and whom I have given this alias, because his name, when fully spelled out, would fill more than an entire page, is a practicing physician in Kuala Lumpur. If you would like to contact him, please email him at: info@KatharinaBachman.de

Sources / Links

Medical Resource Material, the foundation of Dr. K.S.' Treatment:
"Disease Prevention and Treatment" – 130 Evidence-Based Protocols to Combat the Disease of Aging, Life-Extension (Based on Thousands of Scientific Articles and the Clinical Experience of Physicians from Around the World) ISBN:978-0-9658777-8-7
"The Hormone Handbook", Thierry Hertoghe, MD ISBN: 978-2-9599713-5-8
"Atlas of Endocrinology of Hormone Therapy", Thierry Hertoghe, MD ISBN: 978-2-9599713-6-5
"One Man's Food is Someone Else's Poison" Adam Richards, James D'Adamo, Dr. James L. D'Adamo ISBN: 978-0-399-90092-1
"Just an Ounce of Prevention. Is Worth a Pound of Cure", Dr. James L. D'Adamo, Louise Hay ISBN: 978-1-4019-2719-6
"Eat Right For Your Type", Dr. Peter D'Adamo www.dadamo.com/dadamo.htm

Links for ...
Amaranth http://www.naturkost.de/schrotundkorn/2000/sk0012e1htm
Biothemen e.g. Chia Seeds, Omega-3 / Omega-6 Fatty Acids etc. www.biothemen.de
Bladder Wrack http://.4blutgruppen.de/geschenk-aus-dem-eer-fucus-blasentang/
Blood Type Nutrition www.simplify.de/die-themen/gesundheit/gesunde-ernaehrung/einzelansicht/article/ernaehrung-nach-blutgruppen-gesunde-ernaehrung-durch-die-blutgruppen-diaet/
Chilli Pepper http://www.biaschili.com/143/chili-scharf-gesund/
Cholesterol and Eggs http://www.gesundheitsfrage.net/frage/jeden-tag-drei-eier-zu-viel-oder
Chlorophyll http://www.marythemidwife.com/downloads/chlorophyllandblood regeneration.pdf
http://home.arcor.de/gesundheitsmagazin/lifeplus/phytozymepatent_02.htm
D'Adamo Institute www.dadamoinstitute.com
Diabetes International http://www.idf.org/atlasmap/atlasmap
http://www.diabetes-online.de/recht_und_soziales/a/1644779
http://www.idf.org/diabetesatlas
www.diabetesde.org/
Diabetes and Cinnamon blog.nativum.de/2012/08/24/wissenschaftliche-studie-zeigt-zimtextrakt-bei-diabetes-mellitus-erganzend-zur-standardtherapie-hilfreich/
Change of Diet http://www.soziologie-etc.com/med/heilung-o-medi/DrDAdamo/ENGL/blood-group-A/stress-management-A.html
Glutathion www.zentrum-der-gesundheit.de/**glutathion**-spiegel-pi.html

Ketones http://de.sott.net/article/12100-Die-ketone-Ernahrung-Die-vielen-unglaublichen-Vorteile-einer-Ernahrung-basierend-auf-tierischem-Fett-Fur-Korper-Geist-und-Seele

Coconut Oil http://www.coconutresearchcenter.org/article10147.htm
http://www.specialselections.de/coconut-products/alzheimer/

Coconut Water: Substances Contained http://www.kokosnusswasser.net/kokoswasser-inhaltsstoffe-kalorien/

Krill http://wwwcyclopaedia.de/wiki/Krill

Luo Han Guo http://suite101.de/article/eine-suesse-frucht---luo-han-guo-a76387#.VGYjxygRAs0

Luc Montagnier www.houseofnumbers.org/Montagnier_No_Denial.html
www.anti-oxidant-enzyme.com/montagnier.html
http://snoutworld.blogspot.com/2009/12/more-lies-from-brent-leung.html

Melatonin http://www.melatonin-info.net/wirkung.html

Papaya http://www.papaya-papain.com/wirkung-anwendung.html

Phytonutrients http://home.arcor.de/gesundheitsmagazin/lifeplus/phytozyme_patent_02.htm

Plastic Etc http://www.plastic-planet.de/hintergrund_wirtschaftsfaktor.html

Thermogenesis http://www.fitforfun.de/abnehmen/gesund-essen/thermogenese-kurbeln-sie-ihren-stoffwechsel-an_aid_13796.html

Overweight www.spiegel.de/gesundheit/ernaehrung/uebergewicht-2-1-milliarden-menschen-sind-zu-dick-a-972097.html

Acidity www.zentrum-der-gesundheit.de/ph-wert.html

Vitamin K http://medizinauskunft.de/artikel/diagnose/herz_kreislauf/17_09_vitamin_k_gefaessverkalkung.php
http://www.zentrum-der-gesundheit.de/vitamin-k-ia.html

Visceral Belly Fat http://endokrinologie-universimed.com/artikel/vizerales-fett-die-gefahr-lauert-im-bauch

Cells / Nerve Cells: Data http://www-spektrum.de/frage/wie-viele-zellen-hat-der

Recipe Index

KATHARINA BACHMAN, a freelance journalist for many years, has written and published various novels as well as children's and non-fiction books. She emigrated to Malaysia in 2001, where she became editor in chief of a German language magazine. After a several year stay in Dubai, she returned to live in Kuala Lumpur. Since 2006, Katharina Bachman has also been active as cruise ship speaker/ lecturer and Asia-expert for AIDA Cruises. For three months a year she travels the South China Sea, reading from her books and giving lectures on Asian cultures. Her books "SOS - Schlank ohne Sport", "SOS - Schlank ohne Sport.Das Kochuch" and "SOS - Schön ohne Schummeln" are bestsellers to this day. Between March 2015 through August 2017, over 4 million pounds in weight have been lost by German readers alone.

Further information: www.sos-exercise-schmexercise. com / www.katharinabachman.de

Meet the SOS community
Facebook: sos exercise-schmexercise
Instagram: sos-exercise-schmexercise
Youtube: katharinabachman

Meet **Katharina Bachman** personally via social media: https://www.facebook.com/katharina.bachman

Instagram: katharinabachman_sos

Purchase Katharina's products: https://www.vitalingo. com/de/katharina-bachman-edition

About the Translators

Unlike the famous characters in Jane Austen's novel "Pride and Prejudice", Darcy and Elisabeth Powers are not British. **Darcy Powers** was born in Wyoming, USA and grew up in Denver, Colorado. Having travelled to Europe several times and fallen in love with it, at 14, he asked his parents permission to attend an American boarding school in Lugano, Switzerland.

Elisabeth Powers was born in Washington D.C, USA, into a German/American diplomat's family. By virtue of her father's profession, the family lived in several different countries, exposing her to many different cultures and languages well before her teens. At 15, to ensure more continuity in her education, Elisabeth also was sent to The American School in Lugano. It was here that the couple met for the first time and had a brief high-school romance. Having graduated after 2 years, their lives took different directions. Elisabeth went to Heidelberg University to study linguistics, whereas Darcy attended Fleming College to study music in Florence, Italy. He went on to study English literature at the University of Denver, Colorado, where he taught English literature and creative writing. In the mean time, after acquiring her degree in linguistics and translation, Elisabeth trained and worked as an actor in German theatre. It wasn't until 35 years later, that their paths crossed again, rekindling their high-school romance, which soon led to marriage and a new home in Berlin, Germany. At that time, people's perception of food in connection with health was rapidly changing and a flurry of new books on healthy eating habits were appearing all over the world. Elisabeth came across German author Katharina Bachman's hugely successful book "SOS - Schlank Ohne Sport". Not a great gym enthusiast herself, the "Ohne Sport" part in the title (Without Exercise) caught her eye. She decided to change her eating habits and followed the described regimen for a healthier, happier life style, and to spread the word.

Soon many of the non-German speaking friends she told about the book were waiting for it to appear in English, so that Elisabeth contacted Katharina Bachman to enquire. Much to her surprise, the author was not planning on having it translated. Fortunately, soon after their first encounter, Katharina had a change of heart and offered Elisabeth the task of translating the original German "SOS" book into English. Elisabeth happily accepted the offer, on condition that her husband, in his capacity of creative writing and English professor, co-author the translation as a team.

Printed in the United States
By Bookmasters